The Autism-Friendly Guide to Pregnancy, Birth and the Fourth Trimester

of related interest

Supporting Autistic People Through Pregnancy and Childbirth
Hayley Morgan, Emma Durman and Karen Henry
Forewords by Carly Jones, Sheena Byrom and Wenn B. Lawson
ISBN 978 1 83997 105 1
eISBN 978 1 83997 106 8

Women and Girls on the Autism Spectrum, Second Edition
Understanding Life Experiences from Early Childhood to Old Age
Sarah Hendrickx and Jess Hendrickx
Foreword by Judith Gould
ISBN 978 1 80501 069 2
eISBN 978 1 80501 070 8

Stretched to the Limits
Supporting Women with Hypermobile Ehlers-Danlos Syndrome (hEDS) Through Pregnancy, Labour, and Postnatally
Rachel Fitz-Desorgher
ISBN 978 1 83997 249 2
eISBN 978 1 83997 250 8

Parenting When You're Autistic
Tips and advice on how to parent successfully alongside your neurodivergence
Pooky Knightsmith
Foreword by Nerys Hughes
ISBN 978 1 83997 878 4
eISBN 978 1 83997 879 1

Looking After Your Autistic Self
A Personalised Self-Care Approach to Managing Your Sensory and Emotional Well-Being
Niamh Garvey
ISBN 978 1 83997 560 8
eISBN 978 1 80501 699 1

The Autism-Friendly Guide to PREGNANCY, BIRTH and the FOURTH TRIMESTER

Aimee Grant

Jessica Kingsley Publishers
London and Philadelphia

First published in Great Britain in 2025 by Jessica Kingsley Publishers
An imprint of John Murray Press

1

Content Warning: *This book mentions pregnancy, children taken away after birth, examples of poor medical treatment, miscarriage and stillbirth.*

Disclaimer: *The information contained in this book is not intended to replace the services of trained medical professionals or to be a substitute for medical advice. You are advised to consult a doctor on any matters relating to your health, and in particular on any matters that may require diagnosis or medical attention.*

A CIP catalogue record for this title is available from the British Library and the Library of Congress

ISBN 978 1 83997 860 9
eISBN 978 1 83997 861 6

Printed and bound in Great Britain by Clays Ltd

Jessica Kingsley Publishers' policy is to use papers that are natural, renewable and recyclable products and made from wood grown in sustainable forests. The logging and manufacturing processes are expected to conform to the environmental regulations of the country of origin.

Jessica Kingsley Publishers
Carmelite House
50 Victoria Embankment
London EC4Y 0DZ

www.jkp.com

John Murray Press
Part of Hodder & Stoughton Ltd
An Hachette Company

The authorised representative in the EEA is Hachette Ireland, 8 Castlecourt Centre, Dublin 15, D15 XTP3, Ireland (email: info@hbgi.ie)

Contents

CHAPTER 1

Introduction

CONTENTS

Welcome

Hello! My name is Aimee, and I would like to welcome you to this book.

I'm Autistic and have been studying pregnancy and early parenting for over ten years. Since I was diagnosed in 2019, I have been interested in Autistic people's experiences of pregnancy.

Please use the book whichever way is best for you. This means there's no pressure to read it cover to cover, or to start at the beginning. Jump in wherever feels most interesting or important. If you feel that you don't have the headspace to fully read the chapters, feel free to look out for the key points or use the tools.

! If you don't have the headspace to read the chapters, look out for the key bits, which are written like this.

A note on language

Many people in the Autistic community prefer being called an *Autistic person* over being referred to as a *person with Autism*. This is called 'identity first language', and says that being Autistic is an irreversible part of us. Put simply you are either born Autistic or you're not.

You may also notice that I capitalize the A in Autism and Autistic. This is because for me, and some other Autistic people, we use the capital letter to signify the importance of Autistic identities, community and culture.

You may be Autistic and pregnant, Autistic and supporting somebody who's pregnant, or Allistic (non-Autistic) and supporting somebody who's pregnant. This book is for all readers; because of this you will find that I use gender-neutral language throughout. This has been carefully chosen after consultation with a group of Autistic people who had been pregnant. Whilst some identified with traditional labels, like woman or mother, many did not.

Technically everyone who is pregnant is a pregnant person, and many pregnant people will have a partner, family or friend who are supporting them. For this reason throughout the book I'll use **pregnant person**, **partner** and **supporters**. I'll also refer to health professionals; these include midwives, doctors, nurses, lactation consultants (sometimes called an IBCLC) and many more.

How is this book different to other pregnancy books?

In my research, I found that many Autistic people didn't feel that they had been given information about their pregnancy at the right time, or in a way that they understood.

So, I decided to write this book, to hopefully provide information about being pregnant and early parenting in an Autism-friendly way.

This means I use really clear and direct language.

You'll also see summaries of what Autistic people who've been pregnant have said about different parts of maternity.

Why I wrote this book

We know that Autistic people are having babies: one study in Sweden found that over 2000 births in eight years were to those with an Autism diagnosis, and in Wales, UK 0.79 per cent of births (around 1 in every 125) are to those with an Autism diagnosis.

Both figures will be missing Autistic people who weren't diagnosed when they gave birth, or where that information didn't make it onto the computer system. So, there will almost certainly be more Autistic people giving birth. That means that meeting the needs of Autistic birthing people is super important.

A few years ago, I started to look at what we knew about Autistic people's pregnancy and early parenting experiences. I found that there wasn't a book about pregnancy for Autistic parents. I wanted to write a book with lots of things that aimed to help Autistic parents to have a better maternity experience.

This book has been created to be an easy read, with few pages of only writing. I hope that it will be something most Autistic parents will find accessible.

Since 2021, I've done research on Autistic people's maternity experiences. I'm also a founding member of the Maternity and Autism Research Group (www.maternityautismresearchgroup.co.uk). This meant that I felt ready to write this book.

About the author

I've already said hello once, so writing this feels a bit funny, but that's what it's like being Autistic!

So, about me... I grew up in Cornwall, England in a working-class town. I didn't have an easy time at school, and there was lots of bullying. Fortunately, this mostly stopped when I was 16, although I've always known that some of the 'cool' people in most groups I've been part of disliked me enormously.

In my early 20s, I worked as a care support worker for Autistic people in small residential care homes. In the training I had, I heard lots of negative things about Autistic people. This meant that I had no idea that I could be Autistic.

For a start, I had *so much* empathy that it felt painful sometimes. I also 100 per cent knew the answer to the 'Smartie test'. Smarties are small round chocolate sweets sold in cardboard tubes in the UK. The Smartie test was to let a child eat the Smarties in a tube, and then ask them what another child would think was in the tube if it was given to them. Apparently Autistic children said that the other child would say 'nothing' would be in the tube, instead of 'Smarties'. I knew that I would expect there to be Smarties in the tube, so again I felt that I couldn't possibly be Autistic.

Eventually, almost 15 years after I finished that job, I was diagnosed as Autistic. This was when I was in the worst period of burnout I've had so far. It was so bad that around five years later, I've still not regained my ability to walk more than the shortest of distances and I now rely on an electric wheelchair. We'll talk more about the everyday experiences of being Autistic, including burnout, in Chapter 2.

Before I was diagnosed, I worked as a healthcare assistant (nursing aide) on hospital wards, and got a degree, a masters and a PhD. I then started to work as a researcher in 2011 and have done ever since.

I've written two books before. They are to help researchers do their research projects better. This is the first time I'm writing a book for parents.

How do I know the information in the book is good?

I am not a health professional. So, before writing this book I:

- Asked Autistic parents what it was like being pregnant and having maternity care.
- Led a project called 'Autistic pregnancy, birth and beyond: your questions answered' where I found out about the questions Autistic people had about maternity care. The project led to 114 short videos being made by Autistic parents and Autistic professionals to explain different parts of the maternity journey.

There are links to these videos throughout the books – you will need a QR code reader to access them.

You can see all of the videos here:

And there are also a range of playlists on the @AutismMenstruationToMenopause YouTube channel that I run.

- Did a lot of reading from good (trustworthy) places.

In Chapter 5 we talk about how to know if information is good. Also, at the end of the book is a list of lots of good places to learn more about maternity care.

- Had three brilliant Autistic midwives read parts of the book before it was published.

They are Karen Henry, (RM, MA, FHEA), Diane Fox (RM, PGCPSE, PGDPSE) and Rebecca Warboys (RM, IBCLC). Each chapter was reviewed by one of these midwives. They also give their 'Autistic midwives' top tips' in each chapter.

Any mistakes or out-of-date information are my responsibility. If you are ever unsure about something, ask your midwife or health professional.

How to use the book

As I said right up front, there is no expectation that you should read the book cover to cover. There may be some information that you are not interested in, or that you may feel the need to skip and return to when you feel ready for it. It might be helpful to read all of the book, or to get a partner or supporter to read it all, so you are less likely to be surprised (in a bad way) by what happens during your pregnancy.

The book is in three sections: pregnancy, birth and when baby has arrived (this is also called the fourth trimester). In each section there are chapters, headings and sub-headings. There is also an index at the back of the book where you can search for the thing you are interested in.

Chapters 8, 9 and 10 contain birth plan templates that you can use. The full birth plan template is available online and can be downloaded at www.jkp.com/catalogue/book/9781839978609 or via the QR code, along with all Tools in the book, as indicated by a ✸ symbol.

Types of information in the book

As you're going through the book, you will find lots of bits that aren't just plain writing.

These will hopefully help you get the most useful information as easily as possible. They also mean you don't have to read pages and pages of just words!

They are:

Symbol		Meaning
	Exclamation mark	These are really important points.
	Question mark	These are questions that many people have. It can be explaining what a word means, or what happens during a type of test or treatment.
	Script	These are examples of words you can use in different situations.
	Pen and paper	These are tools or activities that you can use.
	Star symbol	You can find these tools on the Jessica Kingsley website.
	Speech bubble	These are summaries from lots of Autistic people about what happened to them.

	Wifi symbol	These are links to videos and web pages, where you can get more information. Most of these are from Autistic parents or Autistic maternity professionals.
	Medical cross	Autistic midwives' top tips. These are included in every chapter.

When I say something that I think is really important, I will say it again with an exclamation mark before it. These might also be useful to take photos of with your phone and show to other people.

Conclusion

You've made it to the end of the introduction. Do feel free to explore whichever part of the book you like next, or go to Chapter 2 to think about the differences between Autistic brains and bodies compared to non-Autistic people, and how these can change during pregnancy.

I always like to hear from people if there are any changes that could be made to future versions of the book – you can find me on Blue Sky @DrAimeeGrant, or via Jessica Kingsley Publishers.

SECTION I

PREGNANCY

CHAPTER 2

Autistic Bodies and Sensory Experiences

CONTENTS

Introduction

Autistic people often struggle with sensory issues, and this can make life difficult. In this chapter we talk about everyday sensory differences for Autistic people, and then think about how they can increase during pregnancy.

These include how we experience the 'five senses' of sight, sound, smell, touch and taste.

I also describe other 'senses' that you may not have heard of, including interoception, proprioception and the vestibular senses – do not worry if these are new words.

We will also explore differences in how Autistic people process pain, which might be related to us being more likely to be hypermobile (including being more bendy).

I then talk about when people struggle to understand or name their emotions, which is called alexithymia.

I then say what happens **before** we get to the point of a meltdown or shutdown, and how stimming can help.

At the end of the chapter, there is an exercise to help you figure out what is causing you sensory overwhelm in your current environment, and how you can try to remove them to make things less painful. There's also a second exercise to help you think about finding more sensory joy.

Common differences in Autistic bodies

There are many ways Autistic bodies are different to the bodies of non-Autistic people. This includes how we experience the world around us, and even how we experience sensations within our own body. These can change in pregnancy, but first we'll look at general differences for many Autistic people when they aren't pregnant.

The five senses

Many people will already know about what are often called the 'five senses'. These are sight, sound, smell, touch and taste.

Autistic people can experience these senses more or less intensely than non-Autistic people.

What does 'sensory avoidant' or 'sensory seeking' mean?
You may have heard about Autistic people being 'sensory avoidant' or 'sensory seeking'. Sensory avoidant means a person is experiencing too much of a sense, and needs to reduce how much they're exposed to it. For example, if someone puts their hands over their ears, they can be trying to reduce how much sound they can hear. Sensory seeking is when someone doesn't feel enough from an experience, so they need to make it bigger. An example would be someone who likes to turn the music up loud to increase the sound they can hear (and sometimes the vibrations of the music). Autistic people can also feel **both** too much **and** not enough of some senses. For instance, they may find the sound of a washing machine painful but enjoy going to concerts with loud music.

If we consider touch, it can be that an Autistic person can find some forms of touch intensely painful, but they can actively seek out other types of touch or tactile sensations which they find soothing. This might be hard for non-Autistic people to understand, but it is important to try to avoid painful sensory stuff when you can. If we have too much sensory pain, we can have 'meltdowns' or 'shutdowns' or even 'burnout'. We'll talk about each of these later in the chapter.

Autistic people experience sight, sound, smell, touch and taste differently to non-Autistic people. This can cause us sensory overwhelm and **pain**.

The five senses in pregnancy

During pregnancy, many people (including non-Autistic people) find that their sense of taste and smell change.

Some smells can feel overpowering or even make you feel sick.

Also, hormone changes can make things taste different (in a bad way) or make you feel sick.

There is medication available to help when feeling sick, and we talk more about feeling sick and eating in Chapter 3 (see page 41).

On top of these routine pregnancy changes, Autistic people also commonly get more sensitive to the things around them. This can include touch feeling different and being more sensitive to sound. Some Autistic people find this difficult, but others enjoy the changes.

You can watch an Autistic occupational therapist talk about sensory sensitivity in pregnancy here:

In my research, Autistic people said these sensory changes made them more anxious, uncomfortable and distressed during their pregnancies.

You can watch an Autistic parent talk about their positive and negative experiences of the sensory world during pregnancy here:

What Autistic people said... about their sensory experience in pregnancy

- Being sensitive to smells was the most common issue, with touch and sound also common.
- Some people became *less* sensitive to sensory issues when pregnant.
- People shouldn't worry that they'll have all these sensory issues, as we're all so different, and every pregnancy is different.
- It can be easy to get very worried that difficult things will happen to you, so looking at positive accounts of pregnancy can help to balance this.
- It's important to make sure your needs are met as much as possible.
- Even if you find being pregnant really overwhelming because of sensory challenges, it can be helpful to think

> that pregnancy has a clear end date, so you can get through it.

! Sensory challenges are likely to increase during pregnancy for Autistic people. This can make them feel more anxious.

The extra senses

Along with the five senses, there are some others that are less commonly known: your internal body messages (interoception), external body messages (proprioception) and balance (vestibular).

Please don't worry if these ideas or words are new to you – I only found out about them in the last few years, despite them impacting me for all of my life!

Internal body messages: interoception

Interoception is the way that the brain experiences messages that have come from inside the body.

This can include things like hunger signals, which can either be intense or relatively quiet in Autistic people. If your signals are 'quiet', you won't know you're hungry until you're really, really hungry. You may also find that you get dysregulated, which is sometimes referred to as being 'hangry' (hungry + angry).

Other common interoceptive messages relate to knowing if you need to go to the toilet (for both a wee and poo), knowing if you are thirsty, and if you are too hot or too cold.

Many Autistic people will experience these messages differently (louder or more quietly) than non-Autistic people.

! Interoception is the strength (or 'volume') of messages from inside your body.

Coordination and balance: proprioception and vestibular systems

The way that your brain senses where your body is in a particular space is known as 'proprioception'. We also have another body system that impacts balance, called the vestibular system.

These systems work together in the background (mostly without you knowing) to plan which parts of your body to move to do a particular task. This means that when you are walking, your body is sending signals to your brain to try to stop you from bumping into things or falling over.

Also, if you are preparing food, your proprioceptive senses are extremely busy planning how you need to move your arms and the rest of your body, for example, to chop ingredients and move them from one place to another without hurting yourself.

It's known that Autistic people have more difficulties with proprioception than non-Autistic people. I definitely am one of these, and regularly have bruises from bumping into things. Also, my proprioception is much worse when I am tired.

! Many Autistic people have weaker coordination and balance systems; this means that we may be clumsy or uncoordinated.

The extra senses during pregnancy

Baby moving

From around 16–24 weeks of pregnancy, you will start to feel the baby move. This will continue until your baby is born. These movements can feel like a swirling or fluttering inside your tummy.

Babies will usually have their own patterns of movement. This includes the time of day that they move the most and any activities that you do that they particularly respond to.

What Autistic people said... about how their baby moving in their tummy felt

- Some people loved every time their baby moved.
- Some were reassured that everything is OK, but it was an uncomfortable or unpleasant feeling.
- For some, some movements felt OK, but others were difficult to tolerate.

- Some people found that baby's movements made them feel sick (nauseous).
- Some people hated it the whole time they were pregnant, but still loved their baby.

Occasionally:

- Some people found all movements were uncomfortable or overwhelming.
- Some people felt their internal organs being pushed or moved by the baby and found it very weird.

You can watch an Autistic parent talk about how they enjoyed feeling their baby's movements here:

It is really important in pregnancy to know what your baby's pattern of movements is, as a change can mean that something is wrong, and you urgently need to be seen by your local maternity unit. We will talk more about this in Chapter 6.

When pregnant, some Autistic people enjoyed the feeling of their baby moving. Others didn't enjoy it or found it odd.

Body changes and balance

Being pregnant affects everybody's balance. As your 'bump' gets bigger, most people need to lean back to balance the weight.

Our bodies are designed to do this, but it can give you pain in your lower back.

If you generally feel like you're a bit 'wobbly' or off balance, this may get worse in pregnancy.

You can watch an Autistic antenatal educator talk about some of these body changes in pregnancy here:

What Autistic people said... about body changes in pregnancy

- Some found it uncomfortable when their breasts or feet grew.
- Not everyone had much growth in their breasts or feet.
- Most people said changes to their body happened slowly, which let them get used to it.
- Changes to their 'centre of gravity' and where their body ended could take time to get used to, and some people bumped into things more than usual.

Later in pregnancy, if you start to feel uncomfortable, taking more time to rest or using a belly support band might help. Also, if you feel off balance or in pain, you can ask your midwife to refer you to a physio (physiotherapist) for treatment.

You can watch an Autistic antenatal educator talk about how you can get used to body changes here:

Some other important differences in Autistic bodies

There hasn't yet been enough research to know all the differences between Autistic bodies and non-Autistic bodies. But we do know some things that impact many Autistic people.

Autistic bodies are often bendy: hypermobility

It is more common for Autistic people to be hypermobile, including having diagnoses like Ehlers–Danlos syndromes (EDS) and hypermobility spectrum disorders. One study[1] found that Autistic people were seven times as likely to have EDS as non-Autistic people.

Being more bendy means that Autistic people's connective tissues, like ligaments and tendons which keep bones in place, stretch more than usual.

Hypermobility in pregnancy

Being more bendy can have an extra impact during pregnancy. When pregnant, hormones make the ligaments around the pelvis stretch to accommodate the baby. If you are hypermobile, you may be more likely to experience extra pelvic pain.

If you have pain in your pelvis, you might want to ask a physio (physiotherapist) for advice and support.

! Autistic people are more likely to be hypermobile, or extra bendy, which can cause pelvic pain in pregnancy. Physiotherapy can help with pelvic pain.

Differences in processing pain

Many Autistic people process pain differently to non-Autistic people.

This can include feeling pain from things that wouldn't hurt most people, such as being touched gently.

Our experiences of pain also tend to be felt in a different way. One example is that many non-Autistic people can easily give their pain score between 1 and 10, but this can be really difficult for Autistic people.

Personally, I often feel really sick (nauseous) when I am in a lot of pain. At one point, I had been unable to eat for nearly a week due to feeling so sick, so I went to the doctor to ask for some medicine. It

---

1 You can find that study here: Cederlöf, M., Larsson, H., Lichtenstein, P. *et al.* Nationwide population-based cohort study of psychiatric disorders in individuals with Ehlers–Danlos syndrome or hypermobility syndrome and their siblings. *BMC Psychiatry 16*, 207 (2016). https://doi.org/10.1186/s12888-016-0922-6

turned out I had a severe tummy bug, but I had put it down to unidentified pain.

Understanding how you feel pain, and how you can tell health professionals, is important in pregnancy. We talk about warning signs and complications, including pain, in Chapter 6, and also think about pain and pain relief methods for birth in Chapter 9. If you are worried about pain, you may want to skip ahead now.

> ! Autistic people often process pain differently. Spend some time thinking about how you feel pain, so you can tell health professionals.

Struggling to identify your emotions: alexithymia

Don't worry if you haven't heard of alexithymia; it's not a word that's used much. Alexithymia literally means 'no words for emotion' but it has a wider meaning.

It can mean struggling to identify or process your own emotions, including those caused by issues relating to sensory processing.

For some Autistic people, this means feeling dysregulated, or 'not quite right', but not knowing why.

Around half of Autistic people experience alexithymia. I definitely experience it; this is particularly related to hunger causing me to be extremely grumpy.

> ! Around half of Autistic people struggle to identify the emotion they're feeling. This is called alexithymia.

We don't know if Autistic people have more alexithymia when pregnant, but I think that it could increase. If you find that you're often getting upset or dysregulated and you don't know why, you could try using the tools at the end of the chapter.

Autistic masking

Autistic people 'mask' or 'camouflage' their behaviour. This is a form of self-protection that is often done without thinking (unconscious).

It's something many Autistic people (especially those raised as girls) learn to do as children, to reduce bad things happening to them. For example, copying the way that a popular person acts can reduce the risk of being bullied.

We know that Autistic people mask when they're trying to get medical care, as often health professionals don't react well to Autistic communication and behaviour. This can be things like making eye contact and 'showing' that they are listening, even though it actually makes it harder to listen and remember what is being said.

Many Autistic people told me that they masked during their maternity care, to try to reduce the chance of getting bad care.

Autistic people shouldn't need to change their behaviour to get fair healthcare, but it is sometimes needed, and always understandable if you do mask.

Masking takes a lot of effort. We'll explore why needing to mask can be harmful for Autistic people next.

A bucket of tolerance

Something I often use to describe what it is like to be Autistic is the idea of having a bucket of tolerance.

To do this, we imagine that every Autistic person has a metaphorical (not real) bucket. Something gets put into the bucket each time we have a difficult sensory experience, spend energy 'masking', have difficulty interacting with people and other kinds of stress.

For example, if I wake up in the morning and I haven't had a refreshing sleep, before I even get out of bed my bucket is no longer empty. I may then find that I've run out of a safe food that I wanted to eat for breakfast, adding another thing to my bucket. In the winter, in my house the heating comes on in the morning, and the boiler makes a noise that is very painful for me. My husband likes to have lights on in many rooms, and these hurt my brain. If I do not give my dog his breakfast quickly enough, he may bark, which is very loud and painful. Looking at my bucket, I may have only been awake for an hour but there is already a lot to tolerate, so my bucket is now a quarter full.

Autistic people will start to feel uncomfortable because of having to tolerate difficult sensory things, or other stressful things. As well as using the word 'uncomfortable' we can also call it being dysregulated or overwhelmed.

! When the sensory world doesn't match an Autistic person's needs, it causes pain. We will become uncomfortable, dysregulated or overwhelmed.

Tool: Think about your 'bucket of tolerance'

If this feels too difficult to think of, don't worry – there are more exercises at the end of the chapter that have more detailed instructions.

You may want to think about what is going into your 'bucket'.

- Spend some time thinking about everything that's been painful for you today.
- You might want to write this down on paper or your phone.

Think about how this impacts you.

- Are you feeling stressed, dysregulated or 'not quite right'?
- Do any of these things look like something you could easily change?
- Can you use the list to be kinder to yourself? You are likely dealing with a lot of difficult things.
- If you find it hard to be kind to yourself, can you think about what you would say to a friend in the same situation as you?

When the bucket overflows

As your bucket fills throughout the day, that feeling of being dysregulated will increase.

If the bucket gets filled to the very top, and there is no more room to fit another tiny thing in, there are only two possible things that can happen. The Autistic person does not get to choose which of these they experience.

First, an Autistic person may have a meltdown. A meltdown is an explosive burst of energy; a lot of the dysregulation will leave the body through movements or sound, such as ranting, shouting or pacing.

Second, an Autistic person may 'shut down'. Shutdowns are the opposite of a meltdown, with the dysregulation pushed inside. When an Autistic person has a shutdown, they may be unable to speak, move their body or make eye contact, even if they can usually do these things. At the most serious, they may become completely immobile and unable to control their bladder and bowels (catatonic), which can take days to resolve.

Both meltdowns and shutdowns are Autistic emergencies, and should be taken seriously. Having a meltdown or a shutdown shows that the environment around the Autistic person is not meeting their needs.

Autistic meltdowns and shutdowns are entirely out of the Autistic person's control. The solution is to make the environment around them less painful.

What Autistic people said... about meltdowns and shutdowns in pregnancy

- Around one in every five people had more meltdowns or shutdowns in pregnancy.
- People didn't always know what had 'caused' them (they had alexithymia).
- Some of these came during or after maternity appointments or during birth.

We know that when Autistic people have a lot of meltdowns or shutdowns they are more likely to have 'Autistic burnout'. This is very important because burnout is associated with suicidal thoughts and suicide.

What is Autistic burnout?

Autistic burnout happens when an Autistic person's needs have consistently been unmet over a long period of time.

When in Autistic burnout, Autistic people lose skills that they have previously had. For example, during a bad period of Autistic burnout, I found it very difficult to drive my car because I found the intensity of everything I could see too much, even when wearing sunglasses.

Burnout is something our minds do to protect us which is out of our control. Another way of saying this is 'an unconscious protective response'. This means that the brain knows that the person cannot take any more stress.

Comforting or soothing actions: stimming

'Stimming' is when an Autistic person does something that they find soothing or comforting. It is generally something done in a set way and repeated. It can help us to feel better if we're feeling uncomfortable.

This can be humming a tune, touching something that feels satisfying such as stroking a dog, using a stress ball, or moving their body, such as rocking, spinning or bouncing on a trampoline. Many people also use favourite music, TV shows, movies or video games as a form of stimming.

What does the medical literature say about stimming?

The full name for stimming is self-stimulatory behaviour, which I don't particularly like as I think it sounds like we're talking about masturbation. Another way that psychiatrists talk about stimming is to call it 'restrictive and repetitive behaviour'.

To me, these words sound negative, which is why I prefer to think of stimming as self-soothing. Most stims will be completely harmless, and because of this, they don't need to be stopped.

Stimming may be done without thinking about it (unconsciously) in young Autistic children. Adults around the Autistic child may tell them to stop, even if the 'stim' is harmless. Because of this, many Autistic adults have lost their 'stims', or coping techniques, or may only use them in private.

Stimming in pregnancy and birth

Some Autistic people stimmed more than usual when pregnant. I would recommend that you stim as much as is helpful during pregnancy, to help you avoid meltdowns and shutdowns.

Stimming during birth is even more important, as it may reduce stress and pain. We will think about this more in Chapter 8 (page 188).

What Autistic people said... about their favourite ways to stim when pregnant

- Touching something that feels nice.
- Moving their hands or feet in a particular way.
- Holding a particular object in their hand and moving it in a way that feels nice.
- Using their voice to sing or hum.
- Being in a bath (make sure the water is not too hot when you're pregnant) or swimming pool.

! Stimming is important for Autistic people when pregnant and giving birth; it can reduce stress and help them feel better.

Creating your sensory toolkit

We know that you are likely to have some increases in sensory issues during pregnancy. We also know that some Autistic people find this has a negative impact on their mental health. For this reason, it's important to try to remove some of the painful sensory things if possible.

Sensory audit 1: taking away the negative sensory stuff

Unfortunately, doing a sensory audit is not a one-off. You may need to do one for each place that you spend a lot of time. I would start off doing this in the place that you spend most of your time, which is likely to be either your home or your workplace.

I have ordered the checklist so that the things that impact most

Autistic pregnant people are at the top. It's OK to ignore anything that isn't impacting you.

Tool: Finding negative sensory things

Sensory area	Possible issues	Possible solutions
Smell	Do any particular food smells bother you?	Ask people to change the food or products they use.
	Do chemical smells like cleaning products, air fresheners, perfumes and scented beauty products bother you?	Wear an N95 mask that fits your face well.
Taste	Do particular foods make you feel sick (nauseous)?	Eat your safe foods as regularly as you like; tell others that this is necessary for your health.
Touch	Do any of your clothes feel uncomfortable (including labels), scratchy, too tight or too restrictive?	You may want to wear maternity clothes early.
	Do your shoes feel too tight?	Feet may get bigger in pregnancy; measure your feet and buy bigger shoes; if it's safe, spend time not wearing shoes.
	Does anyone touch you without asking first?	Make a clear boundary: 'Please do not ever touch me without asking my permission first'.
	Is any of the furniture you sit or lie on uncomfortable?	You may find a pregnancy pillow helps in bed, and may need extra cushions or padding on seats.
Sound	Can you hear sounds that bother you?	Sit quietly and make a list of noises, then try to reduce their impact on you: e.g. closing doors, closing windows, moving to a quieter place, using earplugs or noise cancelling headphones.

Sensory area	Possible issues	Possible solutions
	Is there any buzzing or humming from electrical equipment?	Repeat the above exercise.
Light	Does the lighting feel too bright?	Can it be dimmed? Can you move away from the light or wear sunglasses or glasses with coloured lenses?
	Is there any flickering light (or computer monitors)?	Dust light bulbs, check connections in light bulbs and monitors (turn off the power first for light bulbs).
	Are there any distracting shadows or light patterns?	Open or close curtains or blinds. Move so you are less aware of them.
	Are there any distracting reflections or glare?	Find a way to reduce these, or move away from them.

Unfortunately, many of the sensory things in the sensory audit tool may not be entirely in your control.

You may choose to start trying some 'easy wins', that means things that you can quickly change without much effort.

If you need people in your home, or your colleagues, to change, you will need to let them know. In Chapter 4 (page 84), we'll think about changes you can ask for during your maternity appointments.

Script: Asking people to change their behaviour

These are some ideas for words you can say when asking people to change something:

- '(thing) is making me feel sick. Could you please (do other thing) instead? It would make a really big difference.'
- 'I'm really struggling with the smell of (thing). I'm going to move (further away) so I can't smell it so much.'
- 'It's well known that Autistic people have extra sensory challenges when pregnant. (thing) is usually OK for me, but now I'm pregnant it's making me feel (say how you're

feeling). Would you be able to stop doing this until after I have the baby?'

- (somebody tries to touch you) 'Please do not ever touch me without asking my permission first.'
- (somebody tries to touch you) 'Stop, I don't want you to touch me.'

Sensory audit 2: adding positive stuff

Earlier in the chapter, we talked about stimming. Many Autistic adults will have tried to stop their stimming because of criticism from family or peers in their childhood. I certainly know that when I got my diagnosis, I did not know what my stims were, although as a child I often clapped my hands together at times that were seen as inappropriate, including being on stage during a primary school play.

Tool: Adding positive sensory things to your life

It can be really hard to re-find your stims, so don't feel bad if this doesn't work for you straight away. I've been trying to find my stims for several years and now have some, but not lots.

- Find things from your past:
  - Think about when you felt most regulated, or content.
  - Try to remember the things you spent your time doing that you enjoyed.
  - Give some of these a try.

- Try things that Autistic people commonly enjoy:
  - Moving your body – including rocking, spinning, pacing, tiptoe walking (if you have the balance for it). If you're planning to try anything that would be a big change, check with your midwife that it's safe during pregnancy.
  - Using your hands or fingers – flapping your hands, touching your fingers together in different ways, touching things that feel nice.
  - Using your voice – singing, scripting (repeating

phrases), including from favourite TV shows or films, humming.
  - Listening to favourite songs, watching favourite TV shows or films.

- If you want to start small, get something that you can touch or hold in your hand that feels enjoyable:
  - Fidget toys are now often cheaply available, including in bundles that include a few different things, and many can be kept in your pocket.
  - Hairbands can be worn discreetly on your wrist, and rings can be spun.

If you have hidden your stims for many years, or have not stimmed around somebody, they may ask questions or make comments at first.

Script: Responding to comments about you stimming

- 'My Autistic pregnancy book says that stimming is good for me, especially during pregnancy.'
- 'I've been feeling more unwell because of the pregnancy, and doing this helps.'
- 'I find it soothing, and it isn't harming me or the baby.'
- 'Doing (the stim) makes me feel better.'
- 'I can move to a different place so you can't (see/hear) me if you need?'

You may find that at different times in your pregnancy, a particular sensory thing can change. For this reason, you may want to revisit this chapter if you find yourself getting dysregulated without knowing why.

An Autistic midwife's top tips... on sensory issues in pregnancy

By Karen Henry, RM, MA, FHEA

- During pregnancy, you may experience an altered sense of smell. Some women have a stronger sense of smell so that items may smell different or stronger. You may find that food and drink you once enjoyed, such as cheese or coffee, now do not smell the same and you cannot eat or drink them. Your sense of smell will return to normal when you have your baby but may last until your baby is six weeks old.

- Pregnancy can affect the sense of taste. Your hormone levels of oestrogen and progesterone can make the taste buds on your tongue change so that food such as salt and sugar do not taste the same. You might find that food and drink you once enjoyed now taste different. Your sense of taste will return to normal when your baby is around six weeks old.

- In the first 12 weeks of pregnancy, your hormone levels of progesterone are high to help your baby grow. The higher hormone levels can sometimes make you feel sick or be sick because your stomach slows down the digestion of food. Eating smaller amounts of food more regularly, rather than three large meals, can sometimes help. It is important to drink water when you have been sick, and taking small sips of cold water can help. Seek support from your midwife if you are being sick a lot, especially if you feel unwell.

- As your stomach is relaxed in pregnancy, this can affect your bowels and make you feel constipated. This might mean that you go to the toilet less than you usually do, you might feel pain in your stomach, or you might have to strain to get the poo out. It is best to eat foods containing fibre such as fruits, vegetables, nuts and beans and drink water often to help ease constipation.

- Your stomach being relaxed in pregnancy can also cause something called heartburn. This is nothing to do with your heart – but you may have a burning feeling in your throat and upper chest. In later pregnancy, heartburn may be caused by hormone changes and your baby growing bigger and putting pressure on your stomach. In all cases, drinking cold milk or sucking on a mint might help, and medication is also available from a pharmacy. Be sure to tell the pharmacist that you are pregnant.

- Pregnancy can affect balance because the growing weight of gravity in the stomach area means that you may find yourself leaning back to counterbalance your body. This can lead to back pain. The body is designed for counterbalancing because the hormones progesterone and relaxin soften and stretch the ligaments in the pelvis to allow the growth of your baby in the womb to take place.
- If you already have hypermobility or balance issues before pregnancy, you may find they worsen slightly. You can seek support from a physiotherapist – your GP or midwife can refer you to a service near to you which is free in the UK.

Conclusion

You've made it to the end of the chapter! We've covered a lot of different things, but I hope you now understand your Autistic body a bit more, and that during pregnancy the sensory stuff can get more difficult. I've included some tools that might help you to think about your own sensory experiences, and how you can make things easier. Next, we'll think about staying healthy during pregnancy, although it's OK for you to go to whichever section you like.

CHAPTER 3

Staying Healthy in Pregnancy

CONTENTS

Introduction

This chapter starts by thinking about insurance and access to healthcare.

Then, I'll talk a little bit about common concerns during pregnancy. These are: morning sickness, vaginal bleeding, having a urinary tract infection (UTI), constipation and haemorrhoids (piles), things that you should avoid eating or drinking, pregnancy vitamins, medication and exercise.

The chapter finishes by thinking about mental health in pregnancy.

I will also share the experiences of Autistic people from when they were pregnant, which will hopefully make you realize that you are not alone.

In different countries, the advice may vary from what I'm saying, so if you have any concerns, my advice would always be to speak to your midwife or doctor.

! If you have any concerns about your health, speak to your midwife or doctor as soon as possible.

Thinking about your healthcare and insurance

If you live in a country without free healthcare and you don't have insurance (or have high co-pays), it can be very expensive to get basic maternity care or treatment for emergencies. Spend some time looking at your insurance and any other options available to you to reduce the cost of healthcare.

? I'm on a low income, how can I reduce the cost of my maternity care?

- Ask on social media groups for your country.
- Speak to a social worker – you don't have to tell them you are Autistic but they may find out from your records.
- Some hospitals offer financial assistance, where they will reduce the cost of your bill based on your income – they may not advertise this.

- If you receive a large bill, ask for an itemized bill. It will likely get smaller.
- You may be able to get your bill 'recoded' so the cost of your treatment goes down.
- You can ask for a 'self-pay discount'.
- Many hospitals will offer payment plans where you can pay a small amount each month.

A lot of this process can mean making phone calls with someone in billing. Most of the staff you speak to will be empathetic and want to help you. If phone calls are hard for you, ask if you can have an accommodation so somebody else does phone calls for you.

Morning sickness...and your teeth

During pregnancy, four out of five pregnant people experience nausea and vomiting.

Despite the name 'morning sickness', it can last all day.

We don't yet know if it's more common for Autistic people, but sensory issues with smell and taste increase during pregnancy, so you might experience some nausea and vomiting.

What Autistic people said... about morning sickness

- Some people didn't have morning sickness or only had it a little bit.
- Most had some symptoms, including sickness (vomiting), nausea (feeling sick), heartburn and acid reflux.
- For some the nausea (feeling sick) got worse when they were hungry, so eating little and often helped.
- The sickness and nausea could make them feel really poorly and tired, and make eating really difficult (even their usual safe foods).
- Some spoke to their GP or midwife to ask for treatment,

and the medication helped, especially if they'd been feeling really unwell.

- Eating at specific times of the day could be hard – for some in the morning, for others at other times.
- Only eating the things they could tolerate, such as plain food, 'beige' food or fast food, made things easier.
- Eating a small (and sometimes very small) amount in one go and having a break before trying to eat more helped to stop vomiting.
- Morning sickness could happen at all times of the day.

It is very common to feel tired and fed up with morning sickness, so I would advise you to be kind and gentle to yourself when possible. Most people find that morning sickness stops by week 16 (or between weeks 12 and 20), because of changes to hormones, so hopefully it won't be too much longer until you feel better.

Some people find that eating small amounts of plain food reduces their nausea. Ginger biscuits or tea, or anti-travel sickness wristbands are also traditional anti-nausea remedies.

You can watch an Autistic parent talk about their morning sickness that lasted all day here:

'Heartburn', which is a burning or uncomfortable feeling in your throat and upper chest, can happen more in pregnancy.

If you have morning sickness or heartburn, you can speak to a pharmacist and ask for medication. Make sure you tell them you're pregnant.

If you are struggling to keep any food or liquid in your tummy because you keep on vomiting, you should see your doctor or midwife. This is because you may have a condition called **hyperemesis gravidarum**. Your doctor can give you drugs to make you feel less sick, but if you become dehydrated or start to lose weight you may need to go into hospital to have fluids given through an intravenous drip (IV).

We talk about what it's like to stay in hospital and what to pack in Chapter 8 (see pages 188–191).

What is hyperemesis gravidarum?

Hyperemesis gravidarum, sometimes shortened to HG, is severe or excessive nausea and vomiting during pregnancy. Around one to three out of 100 pregnant people will experience HG. If you had HG in a previous pregnancy, or your mum or sister had HG, you may be more likely to have it.

The symptoms are:

- Severe and prolonged nausea and vomiting.
- Dehydration, making you feel thirsty, tired, dizzy or lightheaded, and having changes to your pee (not peeing much, or the pee being dark in colour or strong smelling).
- Weight loss.

Treatments include:

- Drugs to stop you feeling sick (anti-emetics) that are safe during pregnancy.
- Steroids.
- A hospital stay for dehydration, including fluids being given into your bloodstream using an IV. An IV is a soft flexible tube that goes inside a vein. It's normally put into the back of your hand or into your arm using a needle.

Impacts:

- If you lose weight, there is a risk of the baby being born smaller than expected.

- Pregnant people with HG have told researchers that they feel very tired, depressed and anxious. Tell your midwife if you feel like this.
- We don't know about Autistic people's experiences of HG yet.

! If you can't keep drink or food 'down' because of sickness, contact your midwife or GP.

Script: Talking to your GP or midwife about sickness and vomiting

Tell them about the sickness or nausea:

- 'I feel really sick, but I'm not being sick.'
- 'I'm being sick (say a number) times a day.'
- 'I'm sick every time I eat something.'
- 'I'm not able to keep liquid down.'

Tell them how long it's been going on:

- 'I've been like this for (say a number) of days.'
- 'It started on (say the first day, e.g. Tuesday).'

Tell them how it's impacting you and ask for help:

- 'Because I can't keep food and drink down, I'm starting to feel (e.g. weak, dizzy, lightheaded).'
- 'Because I'm Autistic, I'm limited in the range of food I can eat already, and I can't really eat at the moment.'
- 'I think it could be hyperemesis gravidarum. Do you think it could be?'
- 'Is there any treatment I could have?'
- 'Some medication to help with the sickness would really help me.'

Morning sickness can damage your teeth because of the acid in vomit. You should not brush your teeth straight after being sick, as it can damage the enamel. Instead you can:

- rinse your mouth with water
- rinse your mouth with alcohol-free mouthwash that contains fluoride.

It's also important to see a dentist when you're pregnant. This is because the hormone changes in pregnancy can increase the chance of you having problems with your teeth and gums. Some of these problems could impact your baby.

In the UK, you can have free dental care during the maternity period. If you're outside of the UK, it's worth checking to see if you can get free dental care.

What Autistic people said... about caring for their teeth in pregnancy

- Brushing teeth can be hard for many Autistic people anyway.
- Morning sickness could make it harder to brush their teeth because it could make them feel sick or be sick.
- Some people used a water flosser to clean their teeth instead of a tooth brush, and applied toothpaste to their teeth using their finger instead.
- Setting an alarm could help them to remember to clean their teeth if they needed to do it at a different time of day (to avoid morning sickness).

A bit about vaginal bleeding

Bleeding from the vagina in pregnancy can happen for different reasons at different stages. If you have any bleeding, you should be checked by your midwife, GP or early pregnancy unit. This is because it's not possible to know if there is a serious problem without being checked. They may offer you a scan, or an examination of your cervix to understand why you are (or were) bleeding.

> If you have bleeding from the vagina when pregnant, you should contact your midwife or other health professional for advice.

Early in pregnancy, bleeding can be a result of the foetus implanting into the womb, but it could also be the beginning of a pregnancy loss, including a miscarriage or ectopic pregnancy. Having pain in your tummy or shoulder can be a sign of a pregnancy loss that could be dangerous for your health. There is more information about bleeding in pregnancy and pregnancy loss in Chapter 6. There is also a script of things that you can say if you need to phone for medical help (see p. 110).

> If you are bleeding from the vagina **and experiencing tummy (abdominal) or shoulder pain** it can be a medical emergency; you should **urgently** get advice from a health professional.

It is usually safe to have sex in pregnancy, unless you have been told not to by a midwife. We talk more about this in Chapter 7 (see page 133).

Some people who are pregnant will have vaginal bleeding after having vaginal sex. This can be because of a **cervical ectropion**. But, it could be because of another issue, so you should always seek advice from your midwife or local maternity unit. You would usually be offered a scan or examination of your cervix to check where the bleeding is coming from.

What is a cervical ectropion?

A cervical ectropion is when some of the thinner layer of cells from the inside of the uterus have moved to the outside of your cervix. This is a bit like if you pout your lips (as though applying lipstick) and some of the thinner skin from the inside of your mouth can be seen on the outside. Because the inside of the uterus has a thinner layer of cells than the cervix, people with a cervical ectropion can be more likely to experience vaginal bleeding.

Even if you know you have a cervical ectropion, when pregnant, you should still tell your midwife or other health professional every time you have bleeding from your vagina.

In late pregnancy you may have some mucus containing blood, or pink mucus, come out of your vagina. This can be a sign your body is getting ready for birth. This may happen alongside some contractions in your abdomen.

It's a good idea to seek advice from your midwife or local maternity unit, as they might want you to keep in contact or tell you to let them know if you have any particular bodily changes. We will think more about changes to your body before birth in Chapter 7.

Any bleeding in pregnancy is always abnormal, and you should always get this checked by a midwife or your local maternity unit.

If the bleeding is so heavy that you are soaking a sanitary pad or the blood is trickling out of your body (e.g. into the toilet or down your leg), you should phone for an ambulance straight away.

! If you have vaginal bleeding that soaks a pad or trickles out of you, phone an ambulance straight away.

Urinary tract infections in pregnancy

Changes to hormones in pregnancy mean you are more likely to get a urinary tract infection (UTI, sometimes called a 'urine infection' or 'bladder infection').

If you get a UTI, you can be at greater risk of premature rupture of the membranes and premature birth (see Chapter 6, page 118, for more information). Both of these are risky for your baby.

Because of this, your urine will be tested each time you have an appointment with the midwife. We talk more about appointments in the next chapter.

If you notice any signs of a UTI, you should see a midwife or doctor straight away. This means you should **not** wait until your next routine appointment.

What does a UTI in pregnancy look and feel like?

- Very strongly feeling like you need to pee, or peeing more often.
- Pain or burning when you pee.
- A burning feeling or cramps low in your back or tummy.
- Only peeing a small amount at a time, and still feeling like you need to pee after you've been.
- Pee that looks cloudy or has an unusual smell.
- Blood in your pee, which can make it red, bright pink or dark brown.

If you have a kidney infection, you can also have a fever, nausea, vomiting and upper back pain – this is serious and needs urgent treatment.

Urine infections in pregnancy can be dangerous for your baby; seek medical attention if you have any symptoms. Don't wait for your next appointment.

They will likely ask you to give a urine sample (you will need to pee in a sample pot) to be tested, to see if you need antibiotics. If you have a sterile sample pot at home, you could take a urine sample with you to the appointment.

What Autistic people said... about UTIs in pregnancy

- Signs included: needing to pee a lot more than they had a few days before, going to the toilet and nothing or only a little bit of pee coming out, pain when trying to pee and sometimes pain all of the time.

- Some people found they felt really run down, emotional or generally unwell.
- Some people were given antibiotics to take, and it could be difficult to swallow these with morning sickness.

Constipation and haemorrhoids (piles)

In pregnancy, it is normal for your digestion to slow down. This is so your body can get as many nutrients as possible from the food you have eaten. Just because this is normal doesn't mean it's not uncomfortable. This can mean that you get 'constipated' or 'backed up' with poo.

What does it feel like to be constipated?

I couldn't find any research on Autistic people's experiences of constipation in pregnancy, but in general, constipation can include:

- having to strain or squeeze your muscles hard to be able to poo
- after you do a poo, feeling like not all of the poo has come out
- feeling 'blocked up' in your 'back passage' (rectum)
- feeling full, heavy or bloated
- having a pain in your stomach
- cramping in your bowels (felt in your tummy or lower back)
- feeling sick.

There's also research that suggests that Autistic people are more likely to get constipated. If this is true, it might mean that we're more likely to get constipated in pregnancy.

? How can I reduce constipation?

- Drink plenty of water.
- Increase the fibre in your diet by eating things like vegetables, beans and whole grain foods like brown rice or pasta.
- When you feel like you need to poo, go to the toilet as soon as you can. We know that Autistic people might feel the need to go to the toilet more or less strongly than non-Autistic people, so don't feel bad if you can't do this.

Later in pregnancy, you may get 'piles' (haemorrhoids) because of the extra weight of the baby. These are (generally small) lumps inside and around your anus (bum hole). They can make your bottom itchy, and you may see bright red blood from your anus after you poo. The tips on how to reduce constipation will reduce the risk of getting piles.

You can ask a pharmacist or doctor about any creams or treatments you could use, but remember to tell them that you are pregnant.

Things best avoided during pregnancy

Smoking and nicotine

Smoking can be a stim for some Autistic people.

Smoking tobacco when pregnant can be very dangerous for your baby. This includes an increased risk of premature birth, low birth-weight babies and other pregnancy complications. This happens because smoking restricts the amount of oxygen the baby gets, and exposes the baby to carbon monoxide.

Stopping smoking doesn't mean you have to stop using nicotine, which is the addictive bit in cigarettes. The UK NHS advises that using nicotine replacement therapy such as patches or gum, or an e-cigarette will be much less dangerous for baby, as they do not contain the dangerous chemicals found in cigarettes.

If you are finding it difficult to stop smoking, you will not be alone. Your midwife or doctor may be able to provide you with nicotine replacement therapy, or a pharmacist may be able to help. Remember to tell them you are pregnant as some medicines for stopping smoking aren't safe during pregnancy.

E-cigarettes or nicotine replacements are much safer than smoking cigarettes during pregnancy.

What Autistic people said... about trying to quit smoking when pregnant

- If smoking was a stim, it was important to find a replacement:
  - If it was an 'oral' (mouth) stim, replacements included 'chewellery' (jewellery specifically designed to be chewed), sucking on sweets or lollipops, chewing a pen or using an e-cigarette.
  - If it was a hand-based stim, replacements focused on keeping their hands busy, like using stim toys, or doing crafts.
- Some people linked smoking with certain activities or times of the day, so they tried to change those to break the routine.
- Some people used nicotine patches, e-cigarettes or both to get enough nicotine to stop the cravings.
- Some people found that being pregnant meant that they stopped craving cigarettes, or that smoking made them nauseous (feel sick) or even vomit (be sick).
- Other people found it harder to quit, so they cut out cigarettes more gradually, or let themselves smoke one cigarette a day.

Being around other people who are smoking is known as 'second-hand smoke'. When you are pregnant, it can also be dangerous for baby.

Later in the chapter we have some scripts that you can use if you want to change something around you. This might be useful if someone is smoking in your home, or you want to avoid visiting smoky places.

Alcohol and drugs

Drinking alcohol when pregnant can harm the baby, and the larger the amount of alcohol the larger the increased risk of harm. This includes increases in miscarriage, premature birth and low birthweight babies.

If a lot of alcohol has been drunk during pregnancy, the baby can have lifelong complications due to a condition called foetal alcohol spectrum disorder (FASD).

The reason babies can be harmed is because the alcohol can get to the baby through the placenta. Adults process the harmful parts of alcohol through our livers, but babies do not have fully developed livers.

Drugs, including cannabis, can be harmful for your baby during pregnancy. Cannabis is linked with premature birth and there is some evidence of low birthweight babies.

Some Autistic people use alcohol or cannabis to self-medicate because of dysregulation and overwhelm. If you have any concerns about stopping, speak to your midwife or doctor. You may also want to look at the tools in Chapter 2 (pages 32 and 34), which aim to reduce sensory issues in your environment and help you find 'stims' that can reduce feelings of dysregulation.

Some people may have drunk a lot of alcohol or taken drugs before they knew they were pregnant. The advice from the UK NHS is to avoid alcohol and drugs as soon as you know you are pregnant, and to discuss any worries with your midwife or doctor. They would not usually recommend a termination because of this.

! Alcohol and drugs, including cannabis, are best avoided during pregnancy as they can harm the baby.

Food

During pregnancy, it's recommended that you eat a 'healthy diet', including fruit and vegetables, high-fibre food and protein-rich food. This is because it will help your baby to grow.

For many Autistic people, it can be difficult to follow this kind of diet before pregnancy. When faced with morning sickness, increased sensory sensitivities and the need to grow a new human, it can be even harder.

What Autistic people said... about trying to follow a 'healthy diet' in pregnancy

- Many Autistic people found they generally needed to rely on a limited range of 'safe foods' before they were pregnant.
- Morning sickness could mean people didn't really have a choice in what they were able to eat for at least part of their pregnancy.
- Some people said they could only tolerate particular foods in small quantities.
- Smoothies, meal replacement drinks ('protein shakes' or drinks like Ensure) and vitamin pills could help people make sure their baby was getting the nutrition needed. But some people found protein shakes disgusting.
- Setting an alarm could help some people to remember to try to eat.
- The key message was to make sure you are eating whatever you can and not to worry too much about being healthy.

If you can't follow the recommended 'healthy diet', you could try to add in something from it, such as eating one piece of fruit or a portion of vegetables a day. Make sure to wash it first. Or you could add some more fibre (especially if you are constipated – finding it hard to poo). If this doesn't feel possible, just try to stick to your usual diet unless it contains things that are unsafe in pregnancy (see below). If you find yourself struggling to eat your usual safe foods, or you're vomiting a lot speak to your midwife or doctor.

If you can't manage to follow the 'healthy diet' recommended, you could try to add one 'healthy' food per day.

It's also recommended that you don't eat too much during pregnancy. You may have heard the saying that you are 'eating for two' when you are pregnant, but this isn't actually needed. If you find yourself hungry all the time, speak to your midwife or doctor.

Many people have food cravings when pregnant, often including sweet or salty food. Some people have cravings for non-food items. This is known as pica. This can include things like soil, hair, ice and even building materials like plaster. Pica can happen because of missing nutrients in your diet, so if you have these non-food cravings speak to your midwife or doctor.

Food to avoid during pregnancy

The information on which foods to avoid during pregnancy gets updated every few years. The list below was correct in the UK in 2024. If you aren't sure if something is safe, ask your midwife.

? What food should I avoid during pregnancy?

- Some cheeses, including those from unpasteurized milk, some soft cheeses with a white coating on the outside, and blue cheeses.
- Some meat or meat products, including raw or undercooked meat, liver, pâté and game meats including goose.
- Raw or partially cooked eggs.
- Tuna and oily fish can be eaten, but in limited quantities (two portions a week).

Caffeine

Caffeine is commonly found in tea, coffee, cola and energy drinks. It is linked with pregnancy complications like miscarriage and low birth-weight babies. In the UK, the NHS recommends that a small amount of caffeine each day is safe, including one mug of filter coffee or two mugs of tea.

Vitamins and folic acid

If you're trying to get pregnant or you are pregnant and haven't been taking folic acid already, you should start taking it immediately. Folic acid is important as it prevents serious disabilities, including spina bifida. If you are considered to be overweight or obese based on your body mass index (BMI), your midwife may recommend higher doses of folic acid.

Many people do not get enough vitamin D from sunlight on their skin. When trying to get pregnant and during pregnancy, vitamin D supplements are recommended by the UK NHS.

When you are pregnant, you should avoid taking any vitamin supplements that contain vitamin A. Vitamin A is also called retinol, and too much of it can harm your baby. Many multivitamins that you can buy contain vitamin A, so if you are taking a multivitamin you should carefully check the list of ingredients.

You can buy special pregnancy vitamins, which include folic acid and vitamin D, and do not include vitamin A. They are sometimes much more expensive than other types of supplement, and you do not need to buy these.

In some countries you may get free folic acid and vitamin D (you do in the UK). If you cannot afford to buy vitamin supplements, you may be able to get these from your midwife or doctor.

To help your baby's development, during pregnancy, avoid vitamin A, but take folic acid and vitamin D. Speak to your midwife if you're not sure what to take.

What Autistic people said... about pregnancy vitamins

- Pregnancy vitamins were very reassuring when people struggled to eat a balanced diet.
- Swallowing tablets could be difficult, especially with morning sickness, but 'gummy' vitamins could help.

Medication

When you find out that you are pregnant, if you already take any medication you should discuss this with your midwife or doctor **as soon as possible**. This is because some medicines can harm the baby. If your regular medication is unsafe in pregnancy, your doctor will help you to find an alternative.

During pregnancy, if you are being prescribed a new medication, it is very important that you remind the health professional that you are pregnant.

A small number of medications can enter breastmilk. Often health professionals are more cautious about this than is needed. In the UK, the Drugs in Breastmilk Information Service is provided by the Breastfeeding Network and can provide advice.

! During pregnancy, always ask your health professional or pharmacist if a medication is safe to take when pregnant.

Moving your body

Staying mobile during pregnancy has benefits for you and your baby. It is often safe to continue your normal exercise routine, as long as there isn't a risk of your bump being hit or you falling over.

You should listen to your body and reduce the amount of exercise you do if you feel pain, or it makes you feel tired. If you want to start a new intense form of exercise or have any concerns, speak to your health professional and always start slowly.

Some people will join special classes like pregnancy yoga, and this can be a way to make friends with others who are pregnant. If you would prefer not to go to a class you may be able to find resources online. You can ask your midwife if there are any they recommend.

The pelvic floor

During pregnancy, it is recommended that you strengthen your pelvic floor muscles, starting as soon as you know you are pregnant. This can help with supporting your bump during pregnancy and to reduce the risk of leaking pee (incontinence) after birth.

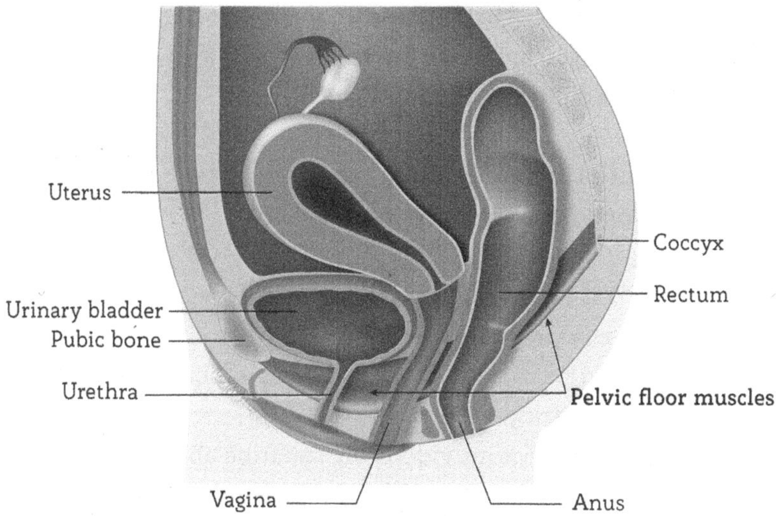

A drawing of the side of an AFAB person's body, including pelvic floor muscles

What is the 'pelvic floor'?

The pelvic floor is something that all humans have. It is a group of muscles which stretch from the front of your pelvis to your tailbone. They form a layered hammock which supports the weight of your internal organs, including your bladder. During pregnancy, they have to hold the extra weight of the baby and the fluid around the baby.

When you are pregnant, the pelvic floor muscles relax, as they will need to stretch during labour.

If you leak pee, such as when you laugh or sneeze (also called 'stress incontinence'), you can strengthen the muscles by doing pelvic floor exercises.

You can ask your midwife for support from a physio (physiotherapist) who can help you learn how to do pelvic floor exercises.

Incontinence can continue after you give birth. If this happens you can be referred to an incontinence specialist.

As an Autistic person, it might be harder for you to identify your pelvic floor muscles, and to do the exercises correctly. I only found out in my late 30s that I didn't know how to tense my pelvic floor muscles when a chiropractor asked me to tighten them and I was barely doing it. If you aren't sure how to do pelvic floor exercises, or you want some reassurance that you are doing them correctly, ask your midwife, who can refer you to a physio (physiotherapist).

What Autistic people said... about pelvic floor issues in pregnancy

- Some had stress incontinence during pregnancy, which could get worse after birth.
- Some had pelvic and low back pain, which could continue after pregnancy.
- Some people found videos on YouTube about how to do pelvic floor exercises, which helped them feel confident to do the exercises.
- Physiotherapy after birth could be helpful, but was invasive (fingers in the vagina) and could be painful, but physiotherapists were usually kind and made sure they had consent.

How do I do pelvic floor exercises?

- Sit, stand or lie in a comfortable position.
- You need to do these two things together, but you might want to practise one at a time until you can do it easily:
  - Squeeze in and tighten the muscles around your back passage (bum hole), as though you're trying to stop passing gas.
  - Draw in your vagina as if you're gripping a tampon or trying to stop peeing (but don't actually do the exercises whilst peeing).
- Once you can do them together:
  - Quickly squeeze and release ten times, working up to 50 times; do this three times a day.
  - When it gets easy to do it quickly, hold the squeeze for up to ten seconds each time; do eight squeezes three times a day.

If these are difficult for you to follow, ask your midwife if they can help or refer you to a physiotherapist.

Pelvic floor exercises may be harder for Autistic people to do, but they're important to stop you leaking pee. Speak to your midwife or a physiotherapist if you are struggling.

Mental health

Pregnancy can be a really stressful time. It is completely normal to feel overwhelmed at points during pregnancy. Common thoughts include worries about money, relationships with partners and family, juggling a new baby when you already have children, and work.

You can watch an Autistic NICU (neonatal intensive care unit) nurse talk about how to cope with anxiety in pregnancy here:

Around 16 weeks into your pregnancy, your baby will be able to feel the sound of your voice, and to recognize it. You may want to talk or sing to your baby. It doesn't matter what you talk to them about as it is the emotion that they can sense; you could share something that you are passionate about to help the bond between you grow.

Autistic people who grew up as girls were often taught to put their own needs aside, and to be polite. This may mean you got used to going along with things that you dislike or that cause you pain. If you like, this book can be your justification to prioritize your own needs. This can mean:

- communicating less with people you find difficult, unless it is required for your job
- not going to places that are painful or difficult for you.

Script: How to say no

I often find saying something positive, followed by a clear reason, helps a 'no' response be heard. If you usually say yes to people, those people may push back against you at first. Keeping your boundary may be difficult, but eventually they will understand.

- Don't answer the phone, but reply by message: 'I'm sorry, I'm too tired to talk right now.'
- 'Thank you for the invitation, but I'm finding this pregnancy hard and won't be able to come.'
- 'That's very kind of you, but I don't enjoy (thing).'
- 'I can't do (the thing they've asked), but would you like to do (other thing) instead?'

If all else fails, 'No' is a complete sentence.

You can also withdraw from people who won't listen to you.

But what if I struggle to speak?

If you find speaking hard, especially if it's when you need to say something difficult, you might find some of these ways of communicating without speaking helpful:

- Because I can find it difficult to speak, and sometimes lose my speech, I have about 30 cards from Stickman Communications (www.stickmancommunications.co.uk) which talk about all of my impairments, and things I'd like people to do or not do (as well as 'STOP', 'YES' and 'NO'). I've only needed to use them a few times, but keeping them in my bag gives me reassurance. You could make your own cards.

- I also have apps (known as 'augmentative and alternative communication' or AAC apps) on my phone that can speak out loud for me when I lose my speech or find saying an upsetting thing too hard.

- I use an Android phone and use Speech Assistant (which is free) most often, as I can type into a box and have my words said out loud.
- I have also used CoughDrop, which is symbol based, but I find it hard to find the words I need quickly, so don't tend to use it any more.
- If my non-speaking times get longer in the future, I will spend time getting better at using CoughDrop, or another similar app like Proloquo2Go (only available on iOS).

- Another 'low tech' way of sharing your needs without speaking could be to write things down for your midwife or doctor, either on a sheet of paper which you give to them, or writing it on your phone and showing them your phone.

What Autistic people said... about mental health in pregnancy

- Pregnancy comes with a lot of big changes.
- They could feel very anxious and overwhelmed.
- Some people felt 'up and down' with their emotions and moods.
- Sleep can be impacted, which could make them very tired.
- Some of these issues could be related to sensory things, like the feel of fabric against their body becoming overwhelming.
- Many people suggested being kind to yourself and resting as much as you can, and doing 'self care' like spending extra time relaxing in bed or having a bath (make sure the water isn't too hot during pregnancy).
- Medication was helpful for some who were very anxious or having regular panic attacks.
- The perinatal mental health team were helpful for some, such as changing regular mental health medication and, were also able to help them prepare for birth with more support.

You can watch an Autistic parent talk about feeling anxious in pregnancy here:

People who have struggled with mental health previously are more likely to have mental health struggles during pregnancy and after birth.

You can help to reduce the stress you feel by doing some of the things discussed in Chapter 2, including:

- stimming
- using other coping strategies you already have; this can include things like watching your favourite TV show or eating safe food
- making the sensory environment around you meet your needs, or if that isn't possible, you can always hide in the toilet for a while
- taking deep breaths.

If you feel like you are struggling with your mental health, speak to your health professional. There are many mental health medications that are safe during pregnancy, and talking therapy may also be able to help. If you feel that you are unsafe, inpatient treatment may be offered, but it often doesn't meet the needs of Autistic people.

! If you are struggling with your mental health, tell your midwife or other health professional.

An Autistic midwife's top tips... on being healthy in pregnancy

By Karen Henry, RM, MA, FHEA

- As mentioned in the previous chapter, pregnancy can affect the sense of taste. Any changes in taste, such as tasting metal in your mouth or having a taste that is not nice in your mouth, may be a sign of something called gingivitis, which can be common in pregnancy.

- Pregnancy can cause your gums to swell and bleed, so in the UK, pregnant women are entitled to free NHS dental care during pregnancy and up to one year after your baby is born. Swollen gums can cause your sense of taste to change.

- Your levels of the hormone progesterone are high in the first 12 weeks of pregnancy to help your baby grow. This slows down how quickly your body digests food and can make you feel sick or be sick. It can sometimes help to eat smaller amounts of food more regularly, rather than three large meals. If you have been sick, it's important to drink water; small sips of cold water might be easier to drink. If you are being sick a lot, it's important to seek support from your midwife, especially if you feel unwell.

- Any bleeding from your vagina must be checked as soon as possible by a midwife or GP. If your midwife or GP are not available, there will be a number to call for urgent queries on the front of your hospital notes. This may say 'Triage' or 'midwifery helpline' or, if you are under 16 weeks pregnant, there may be a number for the early pregnancy assessment unit (EPAU). It is important to have any vaginal bleeding checked.

- Your urine will be tested every time you see your midwife. This is to test for possible urine infections or for certain conditions which may present in pregnancy such as gestational diabetes and pre-eclampsia (high blood pressure). You may be given a small pot to collect your urine in to take to your appointment with you. Catching wee in the small pot can be difficult so you can wee into a jug then pour it into the pot. Make sure the jug is thoroughly clean. If you have any of the symptoms of a urine infection mentioned in this chapter, see your midwife or GP as soon as possible and do not wait until your next appointment. Remember to take a sample with you for testing.

- Women in the UK have free access to a smoking cessation in pregnancy service for themselves and others in the household. Second-hand smoke (being around other people who smoke) is just as dangerous for a pregnant woman and their baby so it is recommended for all in the household to stop smoking. If this is not possible, then ask anyone who smokes to smoke outside, to wash their hands after smoking a cigarette, take off any coats they have worn while smoking and to not smoke in the car. Nicotine and toxins are also carried on the breath and so waiting 30 minutes after smoking to kiss and cuddle the baby is recommended. Further information can be obtained from the Lullaby Trust (https://www.lullabytrust.org.uk/baby-safety/being-a-parent-or-caregiver/smoking/).

Conclusion

You've made it to the end of another chapter! We've covered a lot of different things that can go wrong with your body in pregnancy, from sickness to leaking pee, bladder infections and bleeding. I've also talked about some of the important things to help you stay healthy in pregnancy. I hope this gives you some reassurance, but if you're worried about anything, please speak to your midwife or health professional. Next, we'll be thinking about what happens in maternity appointments, although it's OK for you to go to whatever section you like.

CHAPTER 4

Attending Appointments

CONTENTS

Introduction

In this chapter, we start by looking at your rights during maternity care. The important thing to remember is that you have the right to say no to any treatment you don't want.

Next, we'll look at the different types of staff who do antenatal care. We'll also think about deciding whether (or not) to share that you are Autistic with maternity professionals.

After this, I'll describe the usual timetable for pregnancy care and what happens at those appointments, including the scans and blood tests that you will probably be offered.

The chapter ends by thinking about how you can ask for changes to your maternity care to better meet your needs. This is called having 'disability accommodations' or 'reasonable adjustments'. Many countries have laws that say healthcare services have to make these changes.

Your rights during pregnancy

The really important thing to know is that you don't have to have any examinations, tests or treatments that you don't want to. This is because you have the legal right over your body, including the foetus, when you are pregnant.

Watch an Autistic antenatal educator talk about making treatment decisions in maternity: https://youtu.be/Y5mMvBQxcCA?feature=shared

Despite this, some midwives and health professionals will say things to you in a way that makes it seem that you don't have a choice. This can be because they are in a rush (because there are not enough midwives), but you still have the right to decide.

You should also know all of the important things about a potential test or treatment before you are asked if you agree to have it. This includes knowing about all of the potential risks and benefits. This is known as 'informed consent'.

What Autistic people said... about consenting to treatment during maternity care

- Most people were only given verbal information (not written information) about treatment.
- Sometimes they weren't asked at all before they were examined.
- Sometimes the health professional asked for permission as they were doing the thing.
- Sometimes they were asked to agree to something, but didn't understand exactly what would happen, so they were still surprised – for example, a 'vaginal exam' could involve the health professionals using a speculum to look at the cervix, but also putting their fingers inside the vagina.
- Some people felt pressured by their health professional – for example, if they said they had worries, they were not taken seriously and they felt pushed to do the treatment.
- Sometimes staff listened to their concerns and answered their questions.

You have the right to **say no** at any time during your pregnancy healthcare.

You also have the right to communicate without speaking if needed. This can be using an app on your phone to talk for you, or writing down your questions. You can see more about different ways to communicate if talking is difficult in Chapter 3 (page 60).

How to get maternity care

Once you have a positive pregnancy test, you can contact your GP (primary care doctor) or local midwifery unit. They will be able to help assign you to a midwife and book your first appointment. If you contact your GP, the receptionist may be able to book the appointment for you without seeing a doctor.

The first appointment tends to be around ten weeks of pregnancy.

That's about six weeks after you miss your period. This is because the way pregnancy dates are calculated is from the first day of your last period.

Who provides antenatal care

People with straightforward pregnancies, with no complications, will usually have their antenatal care given mostly by midwives, though you may find that other people are involved.

The colour of uniform worn by midwifery staff in the UK generally reflects their job title or seniority, although this may vary between different areas. You can sometimes find a guide to the colour of uniforms worn in your area online.

It can be hard to tell the seniority of doctors by what they wear. Doctors may wear scrubs (outfits like PJs, which can be washed at very high temperatures) or 'smart casual' clothing.

Who is involved in maternity care?

Midwife: Midwives are specialists in supporting pregnancy and birth. They will have a degree in midwifery and will be registered by a professional body in your country. In some hospitals midwives can specialize in particular areas, including mental health or Autism. Not every hospital will have specialist Autism midwives.

Midwifery support worker: In many maternity services, 'maternity support workers' or 'care assistants' are now involved in giving care. When you are pregnant, this can include things like taking your blood pressure and weight (we'll talk more about this later) before you see the midwife. Once you've given birth, midwifery support workers sometimes provide breastfeeding support. To be a support worker in maternity services you do not need specific qualifications. Because of this, support workers support the midwives and don't independently provide care to you.

Sonographer: The person who does ultrasound scans during pregnancy will often be a sonographer. They are not usually a midwife or doctor. Most sonographers will have some university-level training. If there are any concerns about the results of your scan, a nurse or midwife with extra training or a doctor may repeat the scan.

Doula: Doulas provide support to pregnant people and new parents, including practical and emotional support. They are not midwives, and they usually work outside of maternity services. Doulas have undertaken some training. We talk more about doulas in Chapter 5 (page 103).

Antenatal class tutor: Sometimes midwives run antenatal classes. Other times they are run by people with a range of qualifications; this may include doulas and those working for organizations, such as the National Childbirth Trust (NCT).

Doctor or obstetrician: If you are considered to have a 'high-risk' pregnancy, your antenatal care may be mostly provided by a doctor rather than a midwife. Doctors will all have a master's-level qualification in medicine. Obstetricians are doctors who specialize in pregnancy, also known as obstetrics. Sometimes obstetrics is combined with gynaecology, which is the study of the female reproductive system – then it can be shortened to 'obs and gynae'. Obstetricians will have many years of additional training and qualifications in maternity. If doctors are involved in your birth, you are less likely to have a natural birth without medical intervention.

Anaesthetist: If you are considering a caesarean section (C-section) and have had any complications relating to painkillers in previous surgery, you may be asked to see an anaesthetist in your third trimester. If not, you may not meet them until the day you have your C-section or epidural. We talk in detail about choosing to have a C-section in Chapter 8, and pain relief and what happens if you have a C-section in Chapter 9.

Sharing that you are Autistic with health professionals: pros, cons and how to do it

It is 100 per cent up to you to decide if you want to tell your maternity health professionals that you are Autistic.

Things within hospitals are often not very well joined up, which means that your midwife might not see or have time to read your medical notes.

Even if your midwife has read that you are Autistic, they may not know much about Autism, or they may be short of time, so they might not bring it up with you if you don't start the discussion.

Recent research shows that health professionals (across all of healthcare; not just maternity) don't have a good understanding of Autism and Autistic people's needs. Training for health professionals about Autism is improving. This means that saying you are Autistic should give you more support, not less.

If you have any concerns, you should not feel pressured into sharing that you are Autistic. This is your decision. To help you decide, you may want to think about the pros and cons of sharing your diagnosis, or sharing that you self-identify as Autistic.

What Autistic people said... about deciding to share their diagnosis with maternity staff

- It could be difficult to tell staff, as things felt rushed, so they didn't always feel like there was time.
- Some decided not to tell staff because they feared they might hold negative views of Autistic people.
- Some told some staff when they had developed a relationship with them and trusted them.
- Rarely, people felt that they didn't need to share their diagnosis as they were already getting excellent care that fully met their needs.

Potential benefits of sharing that you are Autistic

Telling a health professional that you are Autistic means that legally they have to make reasonable adjustments to your care, to make it easier for you.

Whare are reasonable adjustments?

In the UK, disability-related changes are required under the Equality Act 2010, as long as it wouldn't be too expensive or difficult for the organization to do them. They are called 'reasonable adjustments'.

This applies to organizations that are providing services, including health services. This means that health services need to make changes so that you don't get worse treatment compared to somebody who isn't disabled.

Not everybody who is Autistic thinks of themselves as disabled. This doesn't impact your rights under the Equality Act.

In other countries there are different laws, but many countries now give disabled and Autistic people these rights.

In some areas, there may be a specialist Autistic pregnancy midwife or treatment pathway. You might be able to find out if there is one in your area by searching on the internet, asking in local mums' social media groups or by asking your midwife.

If there isn't a special Autism in pregnancy service, by saying that you're Autistic you might be able to be seen by the 'perinatal mental health team'. This is a specialist team who support people with mental health conditions. A small number of Autistic people have told me they had maternity care from this team and it was good.

We talk more about disability adjustments at the end of the chapter.

There are some other potential benefits:

- It might make it easier for you to ask for what you need, for example, for them to give you extra time to think during appointments.
- It might make you feel less like you need to hide being Autistic, such as stopping yourself from stimming, or feeling like you

need to 'mask' or hide your Autistic communication style (see Chapter 2, pages 26–31 for more about stimming and masking).

Potential risks of sharing that you are Autistic

Unfortunately, many health professionals have a poor understanding of Autism, and this may mean the following:

- They try to close down any discussion about you being Autistic.
- They make changes based on assumptions rather than what you need; for example, some Autistic parents have told me they felt they were treated like a child.
- Occasionally, Autistic people have reported that maternity staff made inappropriate referrals to social services because of their diagnosis alone. One parent told me they had their child taken away from them for two years because of this.

We talk more about social work assessments in Chapter 12 (page 309). These can happen when you are still pregnant. Rarely, these can lead to the court making a decision that your baby should immediately be taken away ('removed') after birth. If you have any concerns, please skip to Chapter 12 (pages 309–312).

You can watch an Autistic parent share their experiences of child protection and having their child removed by social services here - note this may be upsetting to watch:

What Autistic people said... about what happened when they shared that they were Autistic with maternity staff

- Sometimes it was largely ignored - they weren't asked what that meant and it was never brought up again.

- Sometimes it was dismissed, with staff saying things like 'we are all a bit Autistic'.
- For those who didn't have a formal diagnosis, it could be dismissed because it wasn't yet 'official'.
- Occasionally, midwives helped Autistic people get a diagnosis during pregnancy.
- Occasionally, it resulted in social service referrals just because they were Autistic.

How to tell a health professional that you are Autistic

If you decide to tell your health professional, it might be useful to plan what to say. It may help to think about what you are hoping to achieve before sharing that you are Autistic.

Most people who decide to share their diagnosis will be hoping for at least some changes, or reasonable adjustments, to make their pathway through maternity services easier.

Below are some ideas for words you could use. You might want to write them down or practise them if there is something specific you want your maternity health professional to know.

Script: Telling your health professional that you are Autistic

- 'I'm Autistic and that means...'
- 'I'm Autistic so can you please...'
- 'I'm Autistic so it's important that you know...'
- 'I'm Autistic, so sometimes I behave differently to the average person. I (stim, avoid eye contact).'
- 'It helps me to be able to concentrate on what you're saying when...'

Now we've gone through the basics of who you might meet in your pregnancy care, let's get into what happens in the appointments.

Typical antenatal appointment schedule

The number of appointments you have during pregnancy varies depending on if your pregnancy is considered by your midwife to be low or high risk.

You also usually have fewer appointments if you have had a previous pregnancy where you and the baby were well throughout (an 'uncomplicated pregnancy').

In the UK, if you are low risk you will usually have ten antenatal appointments for your first child, and around seven if you have had a baby before.

Your midwife will be able to tell you, and give you written information, about the appointment schedule in your area.

When you go to any maternity appointments, it is a good idea to take your phone and phone charger or something else to keep you quietly occupied. This is because delays are common. Also, if you need any extra testing, you could have long delays.

! Take your phone and phone charger with you to appointments in case you need to stay longer than expected.

I will now talk about what happens at these appointments, but there may be some variation if you are not in the UK. Most countries have some online information about what to expect during your antenatal appointments.

? What do I search for online to find information about maternity appointments in my country?

- Antenatal appointment schedule.
- Maternity assessment.
- Maternity triage.

If you have any worries about your pregnancy, you should phone your midwife or your local maternity unit, and not wait until your next appointment.

If you are ever worried about your pregnancy, don't wait until the next appointment – phone your midwife or local maternity unit.

You can watch an Autistic midwife talk about what happens at antenatal (pregnancy) appointments here:

Appointment one: 'booking appointment'

You will usually have your booking appointment by the time you are ten weeks pregnant. The appointment can take place at your GP surgery, a children's centre, the hospital or your home. It usually takes about one hour.

In this appointment, the midwife will ask you lots of questions about your health, previous pregnancies and your circumstances. They will also ask you if they can do lots of tests.

What tests will I be offered at the booking appointment?

As standard, your midwife will ask:

- To measure your height and weight.
- To test your blood pressure, using a cuff around the top of one of your arms that is inflated by a machine. It may be a bit uncomfortable, as it can feel quite tight, but it is usually only very tight for a few seconds.
- For you to give a pee (urine) sample, which is tested for signs that you are unwell, such as having an infection or protein in your pee. Sometimes you will be asked to bring a urine sample to the appointment in a little sterile (specially cleaned) bottle that they provide.
- To take some blood, which is tested for signs that you are unwell, including any diseases you could pass on to the baby like HIV and hepatitis, and to find out your blood

group in case you need a blood transfusion following birth.

In some countries, you will be offered a carbon monoxide breath test – you blow into a handheld device. Carbon monoxide is dangerous for babies, and you will be offered advice if your levels are high. This is often due to smoking, being around others who smoke or a faulty gas appliance (boiler or oven) in your home.

You may also be asked if you want some extra 'screening tests' for blood disorders that could be passed on to the baby, including sickle cell disease and thalassaemia.

You can watch an Autistic midwife talk about the different types of tests you will be offered in pregnancy here:

You can say no to any of these tests that you do not want. Also, you can ask for anything that would make it easier for you.

Script: Things you can say if you are worried about testing in your maternity appointment

- 'I've had challenges with dieting in the past and don't want to know my weight; please do not tell me or write it on the part of the notes that I can see.'
- 'I have a history of disordered eating so I cannot get on the scales.'
- 'I'm not able to give you a urine sample today. Could I take a bottle home and bring it back tomorrow?'
- 'I struggle to urinate outside of my home. I'll need to give a urine test next time, can you give me a bottle to take home?'
- 'I'm very anxious about having a blood test. Could I come

back another day (with my partner for support) and have it?'

- 'I find blood tests very painful, do you have any numbing cream available? If not, I can buy some from the pharmacy and come back another day.'
- 'I'm Autistic and find it very stressful to not know what tests will be needed. Can you please tell me what tests I will be asked to have next time?'

The 12-week scan: 'the dating scan' (around 10 to 14 weeks)

The 12-week scan aims to work out your 'due date', or estimated date of delivery, based on the size of the baby.

? What is the estimated date of delivery (EDD)?

The estimated date of delivery is another term for your 'due date'. It means the date that they think your baby could be born. Almost all babies are not actually born on the due date, which can be frustrating as it is out of your control.

The way an estimated date of delivery is worked out is:

1. Take the first day of your last period
2. Add nine months and 7 days

If you know the date of your last period, you can use online estimated date of delivery calculators, such as the one provided by the UK NHS (www.nhs.uk/pregnancy/finding-out/due-date-calculator).

If you don't know the date of your last period, speak to your midwife.

When you have your 12-week scan, they will measure the foetus and give you an updated estimated date of delivery. This is based on the expected growth of the baby.

Health professionals will always use the updated estimated date of delivery from your scan, even if you know the exact date your baby was conceived on.

There is no evidence of any risk to you or your baby from having an ultrasound scan, but it can feel a bit uncomfortable. So you might want to prepare for the scan in advance.

? What should I think about to prepare for my ultrasound scan?

- You may want to take somebody with you for your scans because sometimes you can be given bad news.
- Children aren't usually allowed in the room whilst you have your scan.
- You will need your tummy to be bare during the scan, so it may be easier to not wear a dress or jumpsuit.
- You may need to have a full bladder before doing the scan; you will normally be told this before your appointment.
- It can feel uncomfortable to have the scan, so you may want a fidget toy to hold in your hand during the scan, or to hold the hand of a support person if you have one with you.
- During the scan, you will be able to hear baby's heartbeat. Some Autistic people say that this feels very loud, so you may want to take some earplugs or noise cancelling headphones if you are very sensitive to sound.
- You may be able to buy a picture of your scan. Check with your midwife to find out what happens in your hospital – you may need to take the exact amount of money.

? What happens during an ultrasound scan?

- The person who does your scan will not usually be your midwife, and you may see a different sonographer every time.
- You will usually be in a room with just you, your partner or support person (if you bring one) and the sonographer.
- The room is often quite dark, so the sonographer can see

the computer screen better. You may be able to see the screen, but it may be angled away from you.

- You will be asked to lie down on a medical couch; there will often be tissue paper over the couch, which can feel a bit scratchy.
- You will need your bump to be exposed (so they can see your skin).
- Beside the couch there is usually a computer and a stool for the sonographer to sit on.
- The sonographer will put some gel onto your bump. Some Autistic people find this unpleasant because it is cold or wet. If you prefer more control, you could ask to put the gel on yourself.
- The sonographer will then use a probe which they will push against your tummy. Some Autistic people find this pressure feels quite firm or uncomfortable. The sonographer needs to be quite firm to allow a picture of your baby to be seen.
- During the scan, the sonographer will be concentrating, so they may have quite a serious face, but this doesn't mean that there is anything wrong.
- If the sonographer can't see every part of the baby that they need to, they may ask you to go for a walk (to encourage the baby to change position) and come back, or to come back on another day.

You can watch an Autistic midwife talk about what happens during an ultrasound scan of your tummy here:

During the appointment, you may be offered another scan by somebody with more experience if the sonographer sees anything unusual to do with your pregnancy. This includes if they think you are expecting twins or have any concerns about the baby's growth. The extra scan might be on the same day or it might mean coming back on another day or having extra scans during your pregnancy.

What Autistic people said... about having ultrasound scans

- Waiting to have the first scan could feel like a very long time after seeing a positive pregnancy test – some people paid to have a private scan to get reassurance.
- The gel can feel unpleasant when it goes on your tummy because it can feel cold or slimy.
- The pressure they use with the probe can feel a bit uncomfortable.
- The noise of the baby's heartbeat can feel uncomfortably loud for some.
- Seeing the baby on the monitor or hearing their heartbeat for the first time can make the pregnancy feel very real, and can be an emotional experience.
- Later in pregnancy, scans could be very reassuring to see that the baby is growing.

Extra screening tests (around 10 to 14 weeks)

In the UK, you will also be offered testing to see if you are at risk for Down syndrome, Edwards' syndrome and Patau's syndrome between 10 to 14 weeks of pregnancy.

This test involves an extra blood test when you have your 12-week scan, and the sonographer taking some extra measurements of your baby's neck.

If the results are unclear, or if your baby is high risk for one of the syndromes, extra testing will be needed to know for sure. You will be offered the chance to talk to a specialist screening midwife or doctor to help you decide if you want these extra tests.

Antenatal appointments (after the booking appointment)

The exact timing of the rest of your antenatal appointments may vary depending on what country you are in and if you have had a straight-forward ('uncomplicated') pregnancy before where you and the baby were well throughout.

In most appointments, they will want to test your blood pressure and urine and you may be offered routine blood tests.

Midwives and doctors will also ask you questions about your health, including healthy eating and exercise.

These appointments are also your chance to ask any questions you have. You may not be directly asked, 'Do you have any questions?', so you may need to find an opportunity to ask, or you might find that the appointment is over after what you thought was the small-talk section.

If you have questions about your pregnancy, write them down and take them to your appointment.

What Autistic people said... about their antenatal (maternity) appointments

- Waiting rooms could be busy and crowded.
- Sometimes you had to wait beyond your appointment time.
- Being in the hospital was often difficult because it was busy, loud and bright.
- Needing to wait to hear your name being called meant people couldn't use noise cancelling headphones, and they felt anxious that they might have been missed.
- Appointments could feel rushed and some people felt like they weren't being listened to, as midwives were completing paperwork during the appointment.
- Taking someone with them helped it feel less overwhelming, and sometimes this person spoke on their behalf.

- Some people saw specialist midwives, mostly from mental health teams, and found that they had more time available in appointments and were better able to meet their needs.

Around **20 weeks** into your pregnancy, your midwife will start asking you about your baby's movements, and the sort of pattern they fit into.

Every baby will have its own unique pattern of moving, and it is important to get to know what is normal for your baby. This is because if a baby changes its pattern of movements, it can be a sign that something is wrong.

Many people whose babies died late in their pregnancy later said that the baby's movements had changed before, such as slowing down, being less frequent or stopping altogether. If your baby's movements change, you need to be checked at your local maternity unit. Midwives prefer you to phone them, or the maternity unit if they don't answer, as soon as you think there has been a change. We talk more about warning signs and pregnancy loss in Chapter 6.

? Will the midwife listen to baby's heartbeat?

Midwives used to listen to baby's heartbeat in maternity appointments from around 16 weeks, but this isn't done any more.

It was stopped because some parents found it reassured them their baby was well, and then didn't tell their midwives about their baby's movements changing or slowing down (we'll talk more about this in Chapter 6, page 112).

If you want to hear the heartbeat, you can ask for this, but by itself, it shouldn't be used as reassurance that your baby is well.

! If your baby's movements change, phone your local maternity hospital as soon as possible; your baby could be unwell.

Around **26 weeks** into your pregnancy, your midwife will start measuring your bump using a tape measure. This can feel a bit uncomfortable for some Autistic people. This is one way of checking how your baby is growing. If the midwife has any worries, you may be asked to have extra ultrasound scans.

In the **third trimester**, from around **28 weeks** of pregnancy, your midwife may talk to you about your birth, including:

- where you would like to give birth
- if you would like your baby to have a vitamin K injection when they are born (see Chapter 10, page 239)
- how you plan to feed your baby.

You can ask your midwife for written information to take home with you. There is more information about the decisions you have around birth in Chapter 8.

The 20-week scan or 'anomaly scan' (around 18 to 21 weeks)

This scan checks the development of your baby.

They will check your baby's organs like the heart, lungs, brain, spine and kidneys. They will also take lots of measurements, including baby's head, abdomen (tummy), legs and arms. This is to check for any differences in their growth.

It usually takes around 20 to 30 minutes for your 20-week scan.

The sonographer may be able to tell you the sex of the baby, but it might not be possible because of the baby's position. If you don't want to know the baby's sex, tell the sonographer.

If the sonographer has any concerns, you will be referred to see a doctor.

Tests at 28 weeks

Around 28 weeks you will likely be offered more blood tests, including to see if your iron levels are low (you've 'become anaemic'). If it is found that you are anaemic, you may be given iron supplements as tablets or an IV drip into your vein.

What is low iron (anaemia) in pregnancy? Why is it important?

A lot of iron is needed for you and baby during pregnancy. This means that the iron your body has stored can get used up.

If your iron levels are low, you have anaemia. Around one in five people become anaemic when pregnant.

Anaemia can make you feel tired, weak, breathless and irritable. It can also cause chest pain, dizziness, headaches and heart palpitations (where you can feel your heart beating).

It's important to treat anaemia during pregnancy, as it increases the risk of serious problems, like baby being born prematurely or at a low birthweight. You are also more likely to need a blood transfusion (an IV of blood) after you give birth if you are anaemic.

Tell your midwife if you have any of the symptoms of anaemia.

Low iron in pregnancy can cause serious problems. Tell your midwife if you feel tired, weak, breathless, have chest pain, dizziness or headaches, or you can feel your heart beating (palpitations).

Around this time you might also want to start preparing for birth. You could read Chapters 8, 9 and 10 to find out more about what happens. This can help you think about questions you might want to ask. Some questions that might not be obvious are:

- Is there a parking pass or discount available when I give birth?
- If I harvest colostrum (the early form of breastmilk), how do I need to store it so I can bring it to the hospital when I give birth?
- Could I have a room by myself on the postnatal ward?

Asking for changes to the environment, appointments or examinations, and how to do it

As I said before, you have the right to say no to tests, examinations, treatments and anything else during your maternity care.

Another right that you have, if you have told them that you are Autistic, or if you have another disability, is to have changes made to the treatment you receive so it better meets your needs.

You can tell your midwife about anything that makes the appointment difficult for you, including the sensory environment and how they communicate with you.

If you find appointments very difficult, you may want to contact your local maternity hospital (by phone or email) before your first appointment (the 'booking appointment') to see if they can make changes. If they can't do that, you could ask if that appointment can be done at your home.

Maternity staff should make changes for you if it is possible.

If you find that you struggle to remember things, you could ask for permission to record the appointment. You can use most smartphones to record audio. If you plan to ask for this, make sure you know how to use your phone to record before the appointment.

If you have been told 'no' to adjustments that you really feel you need, you can ask for an appointment with the head of midwifery (the midwife in charge of the unit).

You can also ask to change midwife if you don't feel like there is a good fit with your midwife.

What Autistic people said... about asking for changes ('reasonable adjustments') to their care

- Small adjustments were often agreed to, like letting them put the gel on their own tummy for a scan, or turning off the lights in a room that had natural light from a window.
- Sometimes things were agreed to and done in one appointment but forgotten next time.
- Often, they received a 'no' to bigger changes but when they got very upset and cried about it, it was sometimes reconsidered.
- Having somebody (partner, parent, friend or doula) advocate for them could help get changes to their care.
- Sometimes changes couldn't be made because of

> availability – for example, people needing to stay in hospital because they were unwell during pregnancy couldn't always have a room by themselves.

It can be hard to pick out individual things that make appointments difficult for you, so you may want to look at the tool below to help think about what is painful, and some potential solutions.

Tool: What makes health appointments difficult for you?

Issue	Tick
Sound	
Noisy waiting room	
Background noise in consultation room	
Other:	
Visual and light	
Bright lighting in waiting room	
Bright lighting in consultation room	
Visual clutter, like lots of posters or patterns	
Other:	
Communication	
Being able to speak on the phone	
Being able to speak in person	
My birthing partner speaks on my behalf with my permission	
Talking to the receptionist to 'check in' when I arrive	
Being able to process questions I am asked in a normal length appointment	
Being able to think about what I want to say in response to questions	
Remembering what I want to tell you, or ask, needs me to write it down.	
Other:	
Touch	
Being touched without warning	

Being touched causes me physical pain	
Vaginal examinations would be very painful or traumatic for me	
Other:	
Other	
Finding my way around the hospital	
Remembering that I have an appointment	
Remembering the information I was told in an appointment (paper resources or website links would help)	
Remembering the instructions for when or how to seek advice (paper resources or website links would help)	
Other:	

It can be difficult to ask for changes, even if you have an idea of what could help you. Here are some ideas.

Script: Asking for changes in how your health professional communicates

- 'I am Autistic and need extra processing time. Can you please pause between each thing you say?'
- 'I'm Autistic and struggle to remember things; would you mind if I recorded this appointment on my phone?'
- 'Please can you write down a summary of the information you've given me today?'
- 'I need a written summary so that I have time to think about what we've discussed today.'
- 'Can you please write down everything that I need to do after this appointment?'
- 'Can you please write down the decisions I need to make?'
- 'Can you please write down what symptoms I need to tell you about before my next appointment?'
- 'I'm struggling to speak today because I'm Autistic. My partner is here to communicate for me.'
- 'I'm not going to be able to process everything you're saying; can I please phone my partner to help?'

- 'I don't understand what you mean, can you explain it more simply?'

You can also communicate without speaking if that is easier for you. This can be writing things down or using apps on your phone to speak for you. There is more information about this in the section 'But what if I struggle to speak?' in Chapter 3 (page 60).

How can I support someone during appointments?

This chapter has mostly focused on the Autistic pregnant person. If you support an Autistic person and are going along to an appointment with them, you can be a big help by making sure the appointment is OK for them.

? I'm going to maternity appointments with an Autistic person. What can I do to help?

Ask them about this before the appointment (maybe a week before), so you have plenty of time to make a plan. You could ask them:

- Is there anything you want me to do when we're waiting?
  - Ask for a quieter place to wait.
  - Make sure I listen for your name to be called.
  - Distract you by talking about something you like.

- Is there anything you want me to do during the appointment?
  - Would you like me to take notes?
  - Would you like me to tell the health professional anything you would find hard to say?
  - Are there any tests or treatment you definitely don't want to have? Do you want me to back you up on this if the health professional tries to convince you?

- Is there anything you want me to do after the appointment?

- Would you like me to send you an online diary invite for your next appointment, or send you reminders?
- Would you like me to remind you of anything you need to do?
- Would you like me to ask you if you're having any of the warning signs the midwife talked about (like bleeding, baby's movements changing – see Chapter 6)? If yes, would you like me to ask every day or less often?

An Autistic midwife's top tips... on going to appointments

By Karen Henry, RM, MA, FHEA

- The booking appointment will be the longest appointment you will have (around 1 hour) and all appointments after this will last around 20 minutes.
- At the booking appointment you will be asked about your medical history and whether certain conditions run in your family. It may be helpful for you to take somebody with you who can answer some of the questions for you if you become tired easily. You can also ask if you can audio record important information or record the appointment to listen to any information again when you are at home.
- You can request a longer appointment if you find processing information difficult and need extra time to consider your answers.
- You will often have your midwife appointments in a local community centre, health centre or children's centre. Your scans will usually be done in the hospital.
- If you find visiting new places difficult, you can search the internet to see if there is a virtual video tour of the place you are visiting to help you visualize where you need to go. You may also want to practise travelling to the place beforehand so you can time how long your journey might be and which is the best route to take.
- If you would like a tour of some of the hospital areas you

may go to, this can be arranged by your midwife. You will be accompanied by a midwife to visit the antenatal clinic, the scanning room, the birthing unit and the postnatal ward.

- When arranging your appointments, consider if there is a time of day you would find easier. For example, do you have more energy in the morning or the afternoon to travel to appointments?
- If you find clinic waiting areas difficult to manage in terms of noise, you can ask if there is a quieter room you can wait in. Or you can request an appointment at the start of the day or the end of the day when the waiting areas may be less busy.
- When you are pregnant, your body creates extra blood to help provide nutrients and oxygen to the baby. Because of this, the number of red blood cells can be at a lower level than you need, which is called anaemia. You will be offered iron tablets to increase your levels. When you take the iron tablet, drink some fresh orange juice with it to help it absorb better. Sometimes iron tablets can cause constipation so the orange juice may help with this too. You may also notice that your poo is black – this is normal.

Conclusion

You've made it to the end of Chapter 4! We've covered everything to do with the antenatal appointments that you will likely have. This includes being able to say no, who will be doing your appointments, what happens in appointments and scans, and how you can ask to make them better suit your needs as an Autistic person. I hope this gives you some reassurance, but if you're worried about anything, please speak to your midwife or health professional.

Next, we'll be thinking about how you can find information and people who can help you during your pregnancy, although it's OK for you to go to whatever section you like.

CHAPTER 5

Finding Information and Supportive People

CONTENTS

Introduction

This chapter focuses on finding information and supportive people during pregnancy, although it's also likely to be helpful when you're thinking about support after birth.

We start off by thinking about dealing with people. This includes deciding when to tell people you are pregnant, the unhelpful comments that people direct at you when they know you're pregnant, and unwanted touching of your bump.

Next, we think about where you can find trustworthy information, including thinking about how to deal with information overload and conflicting information.

We then think about how to find other pregnant people.

Last, I talk about a range of sources of support, including from other parents (peer support) and doulas, who are trained to help you through birth.

Dealing with (unhelpful) people

Sharing the news that you are pregnant

There are no rules about when you should or shouldn't tell people you are pregnant.

Many people choose to wait until after the first trimester (13 weeks), because the highest risk of pregnancy loss has passed.

Once you have told people, you can't 'untell' them. So it may be helpful to think carefully about when to share the news and with whom.

What Autistic people said... about things that helped them decide when to tell people they were pregnant

- Thinking about how supportive people would be; earlier in pregnancy, only telling people who would be supportive.
- Excitement: wanting to share the news with close family and friends, or sometimes everyone.
- Worry about miscarriage meant waiting until later for some, or telling people early if they would want support if it happened.
- Feeling poorly because of the pregnancy and finding it easier to tell people than hide it.
- Some people announced their pregnancy on social media, sometimes with scan pictures, but others waited until after birth, or didn't mention anything at all online.

You can watch an Autistic parent's thoughts about changing relationships with partners, family and friends during pregnancy and early parenthood here: https://youtu.be/CI5DSxglDd4?feature=shared

When you are pregnant, you have rights at work. These will vary in each country, but often you are allowed time off for maternity appointments, and you should not lose your job or be denied promotion.

Even though you have employment rights, there is evidence that employers are more likely to treat people badly when they are pregnant or on maternity leave.

The website 'Pregnant Then Screwed' (https://pregnantthenscrewed.com) contains information about maternity employment rights for people in the UK.

Tool: Who should I tell about my pregnancy in the early weeks?

You might want to think about these questions to help you decide who it would be helpful to tell about your pregnancy. There is no right or wrong answer.

- Would you like anyone to know if you had a pregnancy loss? If yes:
  - Think about who would support and listen to you; you may want to discuss this with your partner.
  - You may want to consider waiting to tell people who you have difficult relationships with, or who you think wouldn't be supportive if you had a pregnancy loss.
- Is there anyone you definitely don't want to know?
- If you only want some people to know, can you trust them not to tell other people?
- Would there be any impact on your job if people found out you were pregnant?

Unhelpful comments and touching

As soon as you tell people that you are pregnant, you will start getting a lot of opinions, on everything from what you should eat and drink to how you're going to feed your baby (in six months time!).

Later in pregnancy when you have a visible 'bump', strangers may also start asking you questions. They may ask things like: 'How long were you trying to get pregnant?' 'When are you due?' 'Is it a boy or a girl?' They may also comment on the size of your bump, and whether they think it is big or small for how many weeks pregnant you are.

Some people will also tell you about their own (or their partner's) pregnancies. In the lead-up to birth, you may hear people's birth stories, including things that went wrong for them, which (understandably!) might be worrying for you.

If this happens, try to remember that just because one person has had a bad experience, it doesn't mean you will. There are also lots of people who have had good birth experiences. You could try searching for 'positive birth story' online.

You can hear about an Autistic parent's experience of 'feeling like public property' when they were pregnant in this short video: https://youtu.be/P5ywbfpOegE?feature=shared

People can be very rude to pregnant people, sharing their opinions and stories. You do not have to listen to them.

These intrusive comments can be really annoying for everyone who's pregnant, but might be particularly hard for Autistic people. Remember, you do not need to listen to unwanted information from anyone (although many people make pregnancy-related decisions with their partner). That said, it can be hard to get people to stop talking.

One way to be ready for this is to pick some responses to use and practise saying them out loud before you need them.

Script: Responses to unwanted comments or questions

Things you might say the first time someone makes a comment:

- 'I don't want to talk about it.'
- 'Thank you, I'll think about it.'
- 'You could send me a copy of the research you're talking about if you like.'
- 'I've done my own reading and decided I'm not going to...'
- 'It's OK, my midwife and I have it all in hand.'
- 'It's my choice, and I've decided to...'
- 'I'm sorry, I don't want to hear about other people's births.'

If they won't stop talking about things you don't want to talk about, you could be more firm:

- 'I asked my midwife about the information you sent me, and she said I don't need to worry about it.'
- 'You've said this already, I've made my decision, and I don't want to talk about it anymore.'
- 'Please stop bringing this up, I'm following medical advice.'
- 'Please stop bringing this up, it's making me feel really uncomfortable.'
- 'I'd rather not see you if you won't respect my wishes.'

As an Autistic person, I know it can be really hard to remove yourself from these kinds of conflicts, thinking that if only they fully understood how you felt they would stop making these comments. Sometimes long explanations might work, but other times they might not, and will continue to cause you to be upset.

If you are finding conflict around your pregnancy and parenting plans upsetting, you may want to try a form of passive resistance known as 'grey rocking'.

What is grey rocking?

Grey rocking is being as unresponsive as possible, whilst keeping yourself safe. You do this by being uninteresting and unengaged. The aim of this is to make the person lose interest (because the conflict is part of what can be driving their comments).

It can look like:

- not sharing information and decisions (e.g. your due date, where you plan to give birth, information from your birth plan)
- reducing the amount of contact you have, by leaving longer gaps between contact (e.g. saying, 'I'm busy this week, can I see you next Friday?' or waiting longer times to respond to messages or return phone calls)
- not showing emotion when something is said
- using (very) short responses in face-to-face conversations
- not committing to a thing (being non committal), e.g. 'Thanks, I'll think about it'
- avoiding eye contact
- not responding to messages or emails that are upsetting.

If you decide to try grey rocking, somebody who is abusive may escalate their behaviour to try to force a reaction from you. The most important thing is to keep yourself safe. If you have any concerns, you can reach out to your midwife, the police or a local domestic abuse organization.

What Autistic people said... about when they tried grey rocking about their pregnancy and early parenting.

They:

- found it difficult not to continue justifying why they were saying 'no'
- recorded evidence of bad behaviour from those they were

reducing contact with, such as taking screenshots or saving voice messages
- looked at the evidence of bad behaviour to remind themselves why they were doing it
- had therapy to process how difficult it is to reduce contact with difficult people, particularly if it was their parents or close family members.

! 'Grey rocking' is one way you can deal with people who won't stop breaking your boundaries.

When you start 'showing' (you have a visible 'bump'), strangers, family and friends may want to touch your tummy. Many pregnant people have said that strangers touched their bump without asking for permission first.

Unless it's a medical emergency (where your life is in danger), nobody has permission to touch your body without your agreement. It is absolutely OK to try to prevent people touching your bump.

! Strangers, family and friends **do not** have the right to touch your bump. It's OK to say 'no'.

Script: Things to say when somebody touches you without permission

It's always OK to block (obstruct) someone's hand when they are trying to touch you (or your baby) without permission.

If they are already touching you, you can try to move your body away from them, or try to get your hand under their hand to push it away.

You do not need to explain why, as they are the ones in the wrong.

Things you could try saying the first time someone does this:

- 'Please don't touch me, it makes me feel (uncomfortable/sick etc.).'

- 'I don't want you to touch my tummy.'
- 'No thanks.'

If they don't move their hand:

- 'Don't touch me.'
- 'Get off me.'
- 'Take your hand off me, right now.'
- 'I do not consent to you touching me.'

We think more about these sorts of issues, and putting boundaries in place closer to birth, in Chapter 7.

Finding trustworthy health information

As well as the comments from other people, you might also see things on social media, or news articles, that say something with a lot of certainty about pregnancy and health.

News outlets often try to put a 'spin' on research, to make it sound more important and exciting. Also, they may have misunderstood important parts about the research. For this reason, you shouldn't trust a news article about pregnancy to be the best information on that topic.

A lot of information in the news or social media *won't* be high quality. By high quality, I mean that it is based on research evidence that involved a lot of pregnant people, or a lot of babies. Also, the research would need to be done very carefully to be high quality.

Some of the information will also have a 'conflict of interest': research on infant formula is often done by infant formula companies, who want to make money by selling you their product.

You may also find yourself googling information in relation to a symptom you have or something you are worried about. Here you can find all sorts of sources of information: forums, blogs, news articles and more.

Having so much information around you – including conflicting information – can make you feel very anxious. It can also make it feel impossible to make a decision.

What Autistic people said... about finding information about pregnancy and parenting

It can be difficult because...

- there is a lot of conflicting information, so it's hard to know what to trust
- sometimes midwives or health professionals tell you something different to what you've read
- if you see two different health professionals, they may say different things.

Also:

- it can be reassuring to do a lot of reading, so you know a lot about the subject
- **but** if you're having a problem with something, it can be hard to work out what your specific problem is.

Before the internet, parents would often only have one or two books or would rely on their midwife for information. For that reason, I would recommend that you use the resources prepared by your country's health service along with this book for Autism-specific information.

These resources will be very high quality: many midwives, doctors and researchers will have spent time looking at all of the evidence (including checking its quality) to decide on what the safest thing is. They will also be updated when new information is available.

If you are unsure of where to find information for your country, the first place that I recommend you search for health information is the UK NHS website.

How do I find my country's health agency's pregnancy information?

You can try using these search terms **all together**:

- area: name of your country, state or province
- name of the health agency

- words about pregnancy: pregnancy, maternity guide, maternity care.

For example, for the UK (area), NHS (name of health agency), pregnancy (words about pregnancy), I would type into Google 'UK NHS pregnancy'.

If you want to read in more depth, the next step would be pregnancy newsletters, apps or books. The Australian (www.pregnancybirthbaby.org.au) and UK (www.nhs.uk/start-for-life/start-for-life-emails) health services have weekly newsletters that you can subscribe to.

Some health services have developed their own books which are free to download online. If a book or app is available for your country, it may be beneficial to follow that one, as your midwife should be giving you the same information.

Where can I get free English-language pregnancy books from government agencies?

- Northern Ireland: *The Pregnancy Book* (www.publichealth.hscni.net/publications/pregnancy-book-0)
- Wales: *Your Pregnancy and Birth* (https://everychild.wales/parent-information-2)
- Canada: *Your Guide to a Healthy Pregnancy* (www.canada.ca/content/dam/phac-aspc/documents/services/health-promotion/healthy-pregnancy/healthy-pregnancy-guide.pdf)
- New Zealand: *Your Pregnancy* (https://healthed.govt.nz/products/your-pregnancy-he1420).

It can be very easy to find scientific articles that will terrify you unnecessarily. This is because often we need more than one research study to understand something. For example, the research might only have been done in one hospital, and experiences might vary a lot in different hospitals, or different countries.

When we have lots of studies about something, we carefully gather these together to find out everything we currently know. This is called a systematic review. These will have summaries, called 'abstracts', at the beginning but even these can be hard to understand.

Finding other pregnant people and parents

Pregnancy is such a massive change that it can be helpful to find others who are going through it at the same time as you.

Pregnancy classes

One way that people find other pregnant people is by going to classes. These can include specific 'antenatal', 'pregnancy' or 'hypnobirthing' classes, which have the purpose of teaching you about pregnancy and giving birth. Some of these might be offered by your health service, with others being provided by midwives or people who have other pregnancy-related qualifications.

These classes can be in person, or online using video calls. Sometimes online classes can be pre-recorded and don't involve any interaction with other parents, so check this carefully if you're doing the class hoping to meet other parents.

Other options include gentle exercise classes that are safe during pregnancy. These include pregnancy yoga and pregnancy aqua-fit (in a swimming pool). They aren't regulated, so it may be helpful to look for information about the person leading the class. When exercising whilst pregnant, never push yourself to do something that hurts or makes you feel unwell without getting specific agreement from your midwife.

Peer support groups: baby cafes, breastfeeding groups

Many breastfeeding groups and baby cafes welcome people who are pregnant. Your midwife should know about what is on locally. You can ask them to give you a list, or to write down the names of the one(s) that they think might be good for you.

Many of these groups will have a social media presence (often a Facebook group). You could ask to join the group, and ask if it would be OK to come along when you are pregnant.

Often it is OK to take a friend or partner along with you if you are feeling nervous, but if you'd be taking a man, it might be best to check first if that's OK.

What Autistic people said... about pregnancy and parenting groups

They can be difficult because:

- they can be very loud and busy spaces
- there are expectations about how you behave and speak to other parents
- you may feel you need to mask in the spaces (forcing eye contact, not stimming, not wearing earplugs), which takes energy
- if you don't mask, people may exclude you from conversations
- topics of conversation can be limited to babies and children, which can feel repetitive and dull
- people may judge how you parent
- you may find yourself in conflict with other parents.

Finding other Autistic parents

Many Autistic people will have had difficult interactions with non-Autistic people in the past. Also, it can just be nice for everyone to communicate in the same way.

For this reason, you might want to try to find other Autistic parents in your area, or online, who can better understand your experience.

How can I find other Autistic parents?

- If you're in the UK, contact Autistic Parents UK, who offer peer support in some areas (www.Autisticparentsuk.org).
- On social media:
  - Search for Autistic pregnancy- (or early parenting-) related groups. At the time of writing, there are excellent Facebook groups for pregnancy and

parenting, and a separate group for breast- and chest-feeding.
- Search for Autistic women groups for your country or area and ask if anyone is pregnant or has recently given birth and would like to keep in contact.
- Search for local 'mums' groups' and ask if there are any other Autistic people who are pregnant. This strategy will likely 'out' you in your community, so you may want to think about how comfortable you would be before doing this.

You can watch an Autistic antenatal educator talk about how to find other Autistic parents here:

Doulas

Doulas are people who provide support to others during pregnancy, birth and sometimes in the weeks and months after birth.

Doulas do not have medical training; that means that they are not midwives.

A doula can help you to think through your options, particularly when thinking about birth-related decisions. They also give you and your family emotional support.

Having a doula is not usually provided by health services, so you may need to pay for this yourself, although sometimes there are free services available for those in need.

In many countries, there will be a national organization for doulas, which will often have a register of those who have done the training. This is the safest way to find a doula, although you may want to look for personal recommendations, especially from other Autistic or neurodivergent people.

What happens during pregnancy if I have a doula?

Many doulas will have different packages of support available. The more times that you see your doula, the more expensive your package is likely to be.

At a minimum, you will normally see your doula at least twice before you give birth. Outside of these meetings, many doulas offer support by email, text messages or phone. This lets you talk about what you would like when you give birth, and any worries you have.

As an Autistic parent, it's really important that these sessions are used to share the extra challenges that you think you may have when giving birth, so that your doula can advocate for you. This might include things like the sensory environment, or that you may stop being able to speak. We think about these things more in Chapter 8.

In my opinion, the most important thing that doulas do is to support you during birth. They are a calming presence as many of them have been at a lot of births, and they may be able to support you in a different way than your partner or birthing partner. They can also help to make it more likely your needs will be met, by having extra time to get to know you and your needs.

An Autistic midwife's top tips... on finding information

By Karen Henry, RM, MA, FHEA

- It can be difficult to know where to go for reliable, evidence-based information because some social media sites or newspapers do not tell the full or correct story. Family and friends may mean well but their advice may not always be relevant to you, or be the current guidance. Your midwife can direct you to reputable sources such as phone apps and websites alongside NHS resources if you live in the UK.

- Your midwife, GP or maternity care provider will always

listen to any concerns or worries you may have in relation to any information you have been told, read or viewed online. Make a note of your concerns and take them to your next appointment.

- You will be given a 'due date' by your midwife, which is an estimate of when your birth may occur. Babies are typically born between weeks 37 to 42, and only 5 per cent of babies are born on the 'due date'.

- It can be overwhelming for some women to be asked by friends and relatives when they are due and can feel pressure if the 'due date' comes and goes. Some women find it helpful to be vague about their due date and offer a birth month instead. For example, if your 'due date' was the 15th of April, you could tell people your baby may be born sometime between the end of March and the end of April.

- In the UK and many other countries, you have the legal right to paid time off work for all antenatal appointments, which includes antenatal classes and unplanned appointments. Your partner has legal rights to paid time off for two antenatal appointments too. All UK work-related legal rights can be researched at: www.gov.uk/working-when-pregnant-your-rights

- Covid can cause serious ill health to pregnant women and babies. Research has evidenced that the Covid vaccination in pregnancy is safe and offers protection for you and your baby.

- If the idea of going to pregnancy classes with other people is overwhelming, ask your midwife about online or one-to-one classes. Some antenatal services are offered by private companies so it is best to check the credentials of the people running the classes to ensure you are receiving evidence-based support.

Conclusion

You've made it to the end of Chapter 5! We've covered lots of different things relating to information and people. First, we thought about unwanted comments and touching during pregnancy and how to respond to it. We then thought about where to find trustworthy information about pregnancy and early parenting. The rest of the chapter focused on people who can be supportive, including other parents and doulas. In the next chapter we'll be thinking about things for you to monitor during your pregnancy that could be a sign that you or your baby are unwell. We'll also talk about pregnancy loss and the tests and treatment that might happen if there are signs that you might be losing a pregnancy, although it's OK for you to go to whatever section you like.

CHAPTER 6

Monitoring Your Pregnancy, Complications and Pregnancy Loss

CONTENTS

Introduction

This chapter is about things that happen during pregnancy that are warnings that something might be wrong with the baby.

This is things like bleeding from the vagina, and feeling reduced baby movements. I describe what might happen if you experience these. This includes some of the questions they might ask and the tests they might do, including ultrasound scans, which can be through your vagina (a transvaginal scan). If you are having serious complications, you might be asked to stay in hospital.

The second part of the chapter is all about pregnancy loss, including what happens in early pregnancy and how this might be different from a loss later in pregnancy. Finally, we think about emotions following loss, and making decisions about trying to get pregnant again.

This chapter may feel hard to read if you've experienced a pregnancy loss or are worried about your pregnancy, so please do reach out to your health professionals if you have any concerns.

Things to monitor in your pregnancy: bleeding and other warning signs

When you're pregnant it's important to keep an eye out for changes that could show that there is something wrong with your pregnancy. One of the reasons for this is that these things can be an early sign of pregnancy loss.

The signs of pregnancy loss can vary depending on how far along in your pregnancy you are. Early in pregnancy, bleeding and pain are the main things to look for. Later in pregnancy, your baby's pattern of movement is also very important. We'll talk about both of these now.

One of the really important things to remember is that maternity units are always open, so if you have any worries, you can always reach out for immediate help.

! Maternity units are always open day and night. If you have any concerns, you should phone them straight away.

Bleeding in pregnancy

Bleeding in pregnancy can be a sign that something is wrong. Early in pregnancy, vaginal bleeding (blood in your underwear) can be a sign that something is wrong. But that does not mean that every time a pregnant person bleeds the baby will be lost.

You can watch an Autistic midwife talk about bleeding in pregnancy here:

If you are pregnant and bleeding, you should always seek medical advice. Tell them roughly how much you are bleeding and if you are in pain.

What Autistic people said... about when they had bleeding early in pregnancy

- It was often frightening, with many people feeling scared, nervous or anxious.
- Expecting that it could be a miscarriage helped some people feel more in control.
- Others preferred to think that bleeding didn't mean they would have a miscarriage.
- It sometimes came with strange cramping feelings, which weren't just in the tummy, but could be felt in the cervix, back and legs. Other people had pains similar to their usual period pains.

If you notice vaginal bleeding when pregnant, you should **always** seek medical advice. This can either be from your midwife, maternity unit, GP or at the emergency department. If you find it difficult to make phone calls, you could ask your partner or a friend to phone them for you, but it's important that you can be there too to answer their questions.

Script: What to say when you phone your midwife or maternity unit due to bleeding during pregnancy

1. Introduce yourself:
   - 'My name is...'
   - 'I'm...weeks pregnant.'
   - 'I'm Autistic.'
   - Briefly tell them if you have had any complications so far with this pregnancy.
   - Briefly tell them if you have had any previous pregnancy loss.

2. Briefly tell them what is wrong:
   - 'I'm worried because I have been bleeding.'
   - 'The bleeding started...' (yesterday, an hour ago).

3. Tell them how much bleeding is happening:
   - 'The bleeding is only a little bit; some spots in my underwear.'
   - 'The bleeding is quite a bit; I'm wearing a pad and changing it every few hours.'
   - 'The bleeding is a lot; I'm changing my pad every hour.'
   - 'The blood is a lot; it's trickling down my leg.'
   - 'The blood is flowing out of me.'

4. Tell them if you have any clots or tissue with the bleeding:
   - 'I have had some (large/small) clots with the bleeding.'
   - 'I think I had some tissue come out with the bleeding.'

5. Tell them if you're also in pain:
   - 'I'm Autistic, so I find it hard to know when I'm in pain.'
   - 'I don't have any pain with the bleeding.'
   - 'I have pain like my usual period cramps.'

- 'I have pain like my usual period cramps, but it hurts more than usual.'
- 'I have a lot of pain' (tell them where).

6. Tell them if you've taken painkillers and if they helped to reduce the pain.

7. Tell them if you have a temperature (a fever) and if you have had feelings of being very cold (chills).

You should try to tell them how much you are bleeding. You could think about if it's a few spots in your underwear or how quickly you are needing to change a pad. If you have to change your pad once an hour or more this is very serious and could be a medical emergency. Another sign of heavy bleeding is feeling the blood flow or trickle out of you.

If there are clots or what looks like tissue coming out of your vagina, this is also important; you could save this in a container to take to the hospital with you, or if you can't find a container, you could take a photo. If you don't know how to describe the amount of blood, you could take a photo of your underwear or pad to show your midwife.

! Bleeding heavily, such as soaking a sanitary pad or feeling the blood is trickling or flowing out of you, **is a medical emergency**. Seek help urgently, such as by phoning for an ambulance.

If you are bleeding and also experiencing pain, it's very important to seek advice as it could be a complication that might be serious. This pain could be in your tummy, lower back or shoulder. You might also have pain that feels like period cramps; this might be more painful than your usual period pain.

You can watch a midwife talk about how much bleeding in pregnancy is too much here:

If you've had a pregnancy loss before, it doesn't mean it will feel the same if you have another one. In my experience some have felt like a bad period, but one was extremely painful with some, but not much, bleeding.

Talking about bleeding in your routine appointments

During your routine appointments, your midwife might ask if you've had 'any bleeding' or 'any spotting', meaning they want to know if you've had any vaginal bleeding. You should always tell them if you've had any bleeding, even if it is only a small amount. If you say yes, they may offer to do a scan or other tests to find out why there has been bleeding.

If baby's movements slow down, stop or change

When you are around 16–24 weeks pregnant, you should start to feel your baby moving. If you haven't felt them move by 24 weeks, you should tell your midwife, who will be able to check your baby's heartbeat.

Some people can't feel their baby's movements easily. This is sometimes because of baby's position or where the placenta is. Tell your midwife if you find it hard to feel baby's movements; they may offer you extra appointments.

Every baby will be different in how much they move. This can be in the way they move and the times of day that they move the most. But each baby will have a pattern in the way that they usually move. You should be able to feel your baby move until they are born.

A change in how often you feel the baby moving, particularly them being less active, can be a sign that the baby is unwell. This could be something like an infection, where it is urgent and important to start treatment – it could even be lifesaving.

Should I count my baby's kicks?

Years ago, it was recommended that people counted the movements they felt when pregnant. This was sometimes talked about as 'counting kicks'. There are still some apps available.

But the UK NHS do not recommend you count your baby's movements.

Instead, they say you should:

- try to get to know your baby's pattern of movements
- trust your instincts if you think the baby has changed from its usual way of moving
- contact your maternity unit if there are any changes.

! If baby starts to move less, or changes their usual pattern of movements, it can be a sign they are unwell, such as having an infection. It can be life threatening.

If you have any of these signs, the best thing to do is to tell your midwife, or the other health professionals who are monitoring your pregnancy, **straight away**. That means even if it's the middle of the night, as there will always be midwives working.

The reason it's important to phone immediately is because research with people who had a stillbirth found that the baby's movements changed or reduced in the days before the baby died.

? If I'm worried about my baby's movements, is it OK to buy a doppler to listen to their heartbeat?

These days you can buy dopplers, which are devices to listen to heartbeats, from the internet.

It's OK to do this if you enjoy listening to baby.

But it is **not a safe alternative** to monitoring how baby is moving each day. This is for two reasons:

- Listening to the heartbeat can provide false reassurance that all is well, when changes to your baby's movements show that they are poorly.
- Sometimes you can hear your own pulse, and not the baby's.

It's **very, very** important not to use a doppler for reassurance if baby's movements have slowed down, stopped or changed. You need medical advice straight away.

If you haven't felt your baby move by 24 weeks, or if your baby's movements slow down, stop or change, **phone your local maternity unit straight away. Do not wait! They are open day and night.**

Script: What to say to a health professional when you're worried about baby's movements

1. Introduce yourself:
   - 'My name is...'
   - 'I'm...weeks pregnant.'
   - 'I'm Autistic.'
   - Tell them if you have had any complications so far with this pregnancy.
   - Tell them if you have had any previous pregnancy loss.

2. Briefly tell them what is wrong:
   - 'I'm worried about my baby's movements.'

3. Describe the change in baby's movements:
   - 'My baby has completely stopped moving. I haven't felt them move since (time and day).'
   - 'My baby's movements have slowed down. I think they started to slow down (time and day).'
   - 'My baby's pattern of movements is different to usual. They're normally very consistent, but it's been different since (time and day).'
   - 'I'm Autistic so I've found it hard to monitor baby's movements, but I think they're different and something might be wrong.'

4. They might ask you some more questions.

5. They will probably ask you to go into the maternity unit.

6. If they don't ask you to go in, but you are worried, you could say:
   - 'I'm very worried about this and I'm Autistic, so I would really prefer to get checked.'

7. If they still say no to you going to get checked:
   - 'Could you please record in my notes that I am worried but that you decided not to let me get checked?'

You can get more information about baby's movements here:

What does pregnancy loss mean?

Pregnancy loss is when a pregnancy ends without a live baby. It is very common, with around one in every four pregnancies ending in a loss.

Most pregnancy loss occurs in the first three months. Because of this, it is normal to be worried in the early months. Some people choose not to tell their friends and family that they're pregnant until after the first three months have passed, but it's also OK to tell people if you want to. In Chapter 5 (page 93), there are some questions to help you think about whether you want to tell people you are pregnant.

Language to describe pregnancy loss

In this chapter, I will say 'pregnancy loss', not 'losing a baby'. Some Autistic people have told me that talking about an early loss as a 'baby' felt uncomfortable for them, and they preferred to think of their pregnancy loss as an embryo or a bundle of cells. For people with later pregnancy losses, some have said that using the word 'foetus', instead of 'baby', felt upsetting. Whichever approach you prefer, you can ask people to respect your chosen language.

In the table below, you can see information about some of the common types of pregnancy loss. This includes describing some of the things that might happen. You might find this upsetting, so it's OK to leave it or to ask someone else to look at it for you.

Pregnancy loss usually happens because of an abnormality in the way the foetus is developing. This means there isn't anything you could have done to stop it happening.

Also, just because you are having symptoms of pregnancy loss, doesn't mean you will have a loss.

? What are the different types of pregnancy loss?

Type	How common?	Can it be prevented?	Symptoms
Miscarriage is the loss of a pregnancy in the first 23 weeks.	1 in 8 pregnancies[1]	Most cannot be prevented. People who smoke, drink alcohol or take drugs have a higher risk of miscarriage.	• Bleeding from the vagina • Cramps and pain in your tummy (it can feel similar to period pains)
Ectopic pregnancy is when the fertilized egg embeds itself outside of the womb (uterus). This is often in one of the fallopian tubes, and it **cannot** develop into a baby.	1 in 90 pregnancies[2]	No. There is a higher risk of ectopic pregnancy for people who have pelvic inflammatory disease, have had a previous ectopic pregnancy or surgery on their fallopian tube(s), are aged over 35 years, had IVF (in vitro fertilization) or are smokers.	Symptoms usually happen between 4 and 12 weeks of pregnancy. • Tummy pain that is low down on one side • Bleeding or a brown watery discharge from your vagina • Pain in the tip of your shoulder on the same side as your tummy pain • Pain or discomfort when going to the toilet (weeing and pooing) Not everybody gets symptoms; it can be found on a scan. **An ectopic pregnancy is a medical emergency and needs urgent medical help.**

Type	How common?	Can it be prevented?	Symptoms
Molar pregnancy is when the fertilized egg is not viable, but implants into the womb and grows. It **cannot** develop into a baby.	1 in 590[3]	No. There is a higher risk of molar pregnancy if you have had a previous molar pregnancy, you are a teenager or aged over 45 years, or you have an Asian background.	Symptoms include: • Bleeding or dark discharge from your vagina • Your bump looking bigger than you would expect for the stage of pregnancy A molar pregnancy may cause a miscarriage, but sometimes it will be found on a scan.
Stillbirth is a pregnancy loss after 24 weeks. Stillbirth can happen because the placenta isn't working properly, the foetus has a birth defect or because of complications in the birthing parent's health.	1 in 200 births[4]	Most cannot be prevented. Taking folic acid and having the flu vaccination can **reduce** the risk of stillbirth. People who smoke, drink alcohol or take drugs have a higher risk of stillbirth.	• Baby moving less than they usually do • Leaking fluid from the vagina, or your 'waters breaking'

1 *www.nhs.uk/conditions/miscarriage*
2 *www.nhs.uk/conditions/ectopic-pregnancy*
3 *www.cancerresearchuk.org/about-cancer/gestational-trophoblastic-disease-gtd/molar-pregnancy/about*
4 *www.nhs.uk/conditions/stillbirth*

Most pregnancy loss **cannot** be prevented – this is because there is something wrong with how the foetus is developing. Pregnancy loss is not your fault.

If you are worried about any of the signs above, you should contact your maternity unit. It is very important to be clear about the thing you are worried about.

What does 'waters breaking' mean, and what if it happens before my baby is due to be born?

Inside your womb, your baby is in a bag, or sac. In the bag is a clear liquid called **amniotic fluid**. It can look similar to pee (urine). The sac of liquid acts as a protective cushion around your baby.

Often when you are about to give birth, the bag will burst, and the liquid will come out of your vagina. This can be a slow trickle or a big gush that comes out quickly.

For around 1 in 11 pregnant people, their waters break before their body is ready to give birth (before they are 37 weeks pregnant). This is called a premature rupture of membranes, or a pre-labour rupture of membranes. This is sometimes abbreviated to PROM.

It's more likely for your waters to break early if you:

- have an infection in your womb
- have had vaginal bleeding during pregnancy
- have had a preterm birth previously.

Script: How to describe your symptoms to your maternity unit

- 'I have unusual vaginal discharge in my underwear that is (describe the colour - brown, red).'
- 'I'm leaking fluid from my vagina (describe the colour and roughly how much - have you needed to change a sanitary pad?).'
- 'I think my waters have broken (describe how much liquid).'

Pregnancy loss without symptoms

Sometimes you may not have any symptoms that show something is wrong with your pregnancy. Instead, issues are found when you have a routine appointment or scan.

If this happens, it can feel very shocking.

The treatment you receive would be the same as if you had experienced symptoms.

Healthcare management: watchful waiting, transvaginal and abdominal scans, blood tests

When you speak to the maternity unit, they will often ask you to come in to be checked.

If they are very worried, they may tell you to phone for an emergency ambulance.

This can be a really stressful time. Whilst you're on the phone, you can check where in the hospital you need to go. It may be the maternity unit, but it may be a special early pregnancy unit in a different part of the hospital. If you don't know the hospital, you could ask for directions or where the closest car park is.

If you get to the hospital and can't find where to go, don't panic. Phone them back and explain you've been asked to come in and briefly tell them the reason, such as 'because I'm bleeding' or 'because I'm 23 weeks pregnant and baby is moving less than usual'.

! If you are asked to come to the hospital, ask them where you need to go. You can also ask them about parking. Phone back if you get lost.

If you're in the UK, you may go to a specialist early pregnancy unit.

Watch me talk about early pregnancy units here:

If I'm having pregnancy complications, what should I take to hospital?

It may take a while for you to see a health professional, so I would recommend taking enough things to keep you comfortable for at least a few hours. You might want to include:

- A phone and your phone charger, book, craft activity or something else to help distract you.
- Anything that might help you be in a difficult sensory environment, such as sunglasses, earplugs or noise cancelling headphones.
- Something that you can stim with, such as a squishy toy or other object to keep your hands busy.
- Food and drink, although if the health professionals think there is a chance you may need surgery that day, you may be told not to eat or drink anything.
- If you think you might find it difficult to speak, you could take some paper and a pen, or use your phone to type things, or use a special AAC (augmentative and alternative communication) app that speaks for you (see the section 'But what if I struggle to speak?' in Chapter 3, page 60).
- You might also want to pack an overnight bag in case you need to stay in hospital. You might want to include:
  - changes of clothes, especially if you are bleeding a lot
  - sanitary pads
  - comfort items
  - comfort food and drinks (although you might not be able to use a fridge on the ward).

! If you go into hospital for pregnancy complications, take your phone and phone charger with you in case you need to stay longer than expected.

When you arrive at the hospital, you might need to give the same information that you already gave over the phone. It's likely that one of the first things they do is ask to check your 'observations', which are also sometimes called 'obs' or 'vital signs'.

? **What are 'obs', 'observations', 'vital observations' or 'vitals'?**

These words all mean the same thing. They generally include doing all of these tests:

- **Blood pressure:** They will use a soft cuff around the top of one of your arms. It fastens with Velcro, and is gently inflated by a machine. It may be a bit uncomfortable, as it can feel quite tight, but it is usually only very tight for a few seconds.
- **Pulse and blood oxygen level:** They will put a small peg- or clip-like monitor or a flexible sensor onto one fingertip (or occasionally your ear lobe). It shouldn't hurt.
- **Temperature:** They will use a thermometer to take your temperature. These may be infrared ones that are held up to your forehead, or digital thermometers that go into the ear.

The health professional may also count how quickly you're breathing. They usually don't tell you they are doing this, as this can make you conscious of how you're breathing.

If your health professionals have any worries about your health, they will ask to do a set of obs to check. It should only take a few minutes.

You may have some blood taken, usually from a small needle put into your arm. This is to test the amount of pregnancy hormones in your blood. In the first three months of pregnancy, this test is usually done twice, a few days apart, to see if the hormone levels are reducing. Reducing hormone levels can mean that you are having a pregnancy loss, like a miscarriage or ectopic pregnancy.

What Autistic people said... about when they went into hospital because they were bleeding in pregnancy

- They understood it was necessary, but still felt anxious.
- The hospital environment could be overwhelming.
- Scans could be helpful, showing either that the pregnancy was going OK, or that it might not be.
- Some people found staff to be kind and helpful; others didn't.

You will often be offered an ultrasound scan. If you are early in pregnancy (up to around 10 to 12 weeks), the person doing your scan may ask for your permission to do a 'transvaginal' (through the vagina) scan. You do not have to say yes to this, and if you say no, they should do a scan of your belly instead. The reason to do the scan through the vagina is they can get closer to the womb, and will be able to see better.

What is a transvaginal scan? What does it feel like?

A transvaginal scan is a type of ultrasound used to look at your womb and the surrounding areas. To do the scan, a probe that is long and slim will be covered with a sheath (similar to a condom), a blob of ultrasound gel will be put on the tip, and then the probe will be inserted into your vagina.

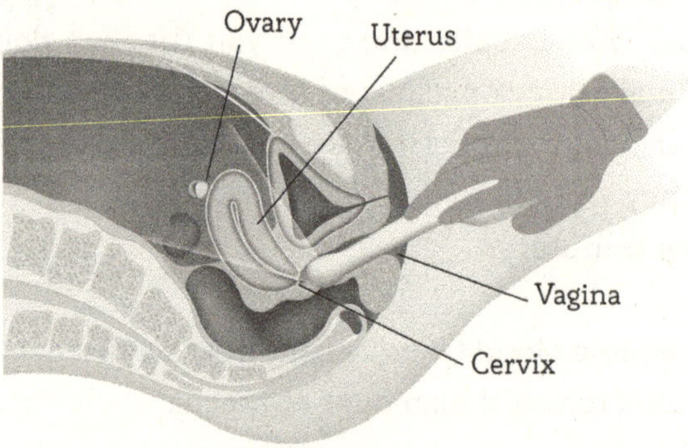

A drawing of a transvaginal scan

I've had several transvaginal scans because of bleeding and pain during early pregnancy. For me, they've always been a bit uncomfortable, but often the nurse or doctor have been really reassuring and told me what they're doing. I have had one experience which was more painful, as the doctor was less gentle when moving the probe around inside me to get the best view.

You can watch an Autistic midwife talk about transvaginal scans here:

Watchful waiting

If you are early in your pregnancy, and not in significant pain, you may be sent home after these tests. At this time, the health professionals may not know if you are losing your baby, as sometimes another set of tests in a few days is needed.

Even if the health professionals know that you are going to lose your baby, they may send you home. This is to see if your body will naturally start to miscarry. This means that without the use of medicine or surgery, you will start bleeding more heavily from the vagina.

Your doctor may ask you or your partner to regularly update them on how you are feeling. This is because if you have an increase in pain, or you start to feel more unwell it could be a sign of a complication. If this happens, you may need medicine or surgery to remove all of the parts of the pregnancy.

Staying in hospital for observation or treatment

If the health professional thinks that you or your baby are quite unwell, they may advise that you stay in hospital. We talk about some of the things that might be difficult when staying in hospital, and what to pack, in Chapter 8.

One of the major reasons why you might be asked to stay in hospital is that people who are having a pregnancy loss can become very unwell quite quickly. Having you in the hospital means that if it's needed, they could get you into emergency surgery quickly.

Being in hospital is often quite difficult for us Autistic people. You may wish to tell the health professionals that you are Autistic, so that you can ask them to make changes for you. You can read more about choosing to tell your health professionals that you are Autistic in Chapter 4 (page 70).

If you realize that you would really benefit from some items being brought in from home, this might be possible outside of the visiting hours on the ward. You can ask your nurse about this.

What Autistic people said... about when they had treatment for a pregnancy loss

- It could feel really upsetting to be losing a pregnancy in hospital, where they couldn't fully be themselves.
- It wasn't always clear what was going to happen and when; some people felt they didn't get enough information.
- Some people felt very upset by the way their pregnancy loss was described by health professionals.
- Health professionals sometimes didn't understand how much pain the person was in.
- Some Autistic people recommend trying to keep calm and get through it, thinking of it as something essential to keep them well.
- Some people said the treatment was so bad that when they had another pregnancy loss, they didn't ask for help.

What happens to your body following pregnancy loss

Before 20 weeks

If you have an early pregnancy loss, the most common type is a miscarriage.

With a miscarriage, you will normally pass most of the tissue in a few hours. You may still get cramping and pain for a day. It is normal for you to have **light** bleeding for four to six weeks. If you are **bleeding heavily, or passing clots or tissue**, you may need treatment to help remove the rest of the pregnancy. The reason for this is because you can get an infection from any pregnancy contents left behind. This can be very serious.

! Anything more than light bleeding after a miscarriage should be checked by a health professional. This is because you can become very unwell from pregnancy contents left behind.

What Autistic people said... about their early pregnancy loss

- Some people found it very upsetting and grieved the loss straight away – this could include being angry, crying or having meltdowns and shutdowns.
- Some people were in shock, and went into 'autopilot' to get through treatment.
- For others it was helpful to think about it as a biological process, and their body doing what was needed to keep them well.

Treatment for miscarriage and early pregnancy loss

There are two types of treatment given for early pregnancy loss.

The first type is medical management. This can involve you taking tablets orally (swallowing them with water), or inserting a different type of tablet into your vagina (a pessary). If you're having an ectopic pregnancy, you may be given an injection. These medicines tell your body to let the lining of the womb come away, along with the pregnancy, through your vagina. This may cause some pain, cramping and contractions.

Usually you will start to pass the pregnancy contents around four to six hours after the second set of tablets. These medicines do not fully remove the pregnancy for everyone, and over one in four people will need more treatment. This can be giving you more of the medication, or advising you to have surgical management.

The second type of treatment is surgical management. You don't have to try taking the medication before having surgery.

If you have surgery, you will not be given an exact time when it will happen. This means you can spend quite a lot of time waiting. Most people will have a general anaesthetic: this means being fully asleep when the surgery happens. You will not be able to eat or drink before this, usually for at least six hours before, but please check with your hospital.

If you are having a miscarriage, you will be given some tablets to put in your vagina before the surgery. This is because the surgery is done through your vagina, by getting your cervix to open.

Watch me talk about treatment for miscarriage here:

If you have an ectopic pregnancy, or some other forms of pregnancy loss, they may do the surgery through your tummy, known as a laparoscopy, making some small cuts to do 'keyhole surgery'.

Watch me talk about treatment for ectopic pregnancy here:

Stillbirth (after 20 weeks)

Despite the name, most stillbirths happen in the womb, they don't usually happen during birth.

If it's found that you have a stillbirth, your health professional will talk to you about the safest way to deliver the foetus. The options are similar to if you give birth to a live baby, including inducing your labour, allowing a natural vaginal birth to happen or a caesarean section. You can read more about these types of birth in Chapter 9.

It can take two weeks for natural labour to start after a stillbirth. Because of this, it may not always be safe, for your health, to wait for a natural birth. If you decide to wait for a natural labour, but find the waiting becomes too difficult for you, reach out to the maternity unit that has been treating you and they will be able to talk to you about your options to start the delivery.

Starting your delivery is also called 'inducing labour' or 'having an induction'. You would be admitted to hospital, on that day or a day you agree on with the hospital staff. To induce you, the health professional may 'break your water' or give you medicine to start your labour. We talk about both of these options in Chapter 8.

During delivery, you will be supported by midwives and health professionals, and they can help you after the delivery too. It is completely up to you how much you would like to see or touch the foetus. The midwives can also help you with making memories, such as photos, and in some hospitals, they may offer memory boxes with other options for keepsakes.

You can watch an Autistic midwife talk about stillbirth here:

If you have a stillbirth, because you have gone through a delivery, your breasts will start to produce milk. You may be able to take medicine to stop this from happening. Some parents decide that they would like to express their breastmilk and give it to a milk bank so it can be given to babies whose parents aren't able to breastfeed. If you would like to do this, ask your midwife for information.

What Autistic people said... about their stillbirth experience

- It could be a very big shock.
- It was hard to make sense of what happened; often there weren't any signs that something was wrong.
- After birth they held the baby, and it could feel hard giving the baby to health professionals when the baby needed to be taken away.
- They could feel very guilty, worrying if they could have done something to prevent it.
- Because relatively few people have a stillbirth, it was hard to find people to talk to who could understand.
- Some people found counselling or baby loss charities helpful; others took comfort in their religion.

- Some were very angry when they thought that the health professionals might have done something wrong, and some of these considered making a complaint.

Termination of pregnancy because of a serious condition

In Chapter 4 we talked about tests that will be offered to you during pregnancy. Some of these are for signs the foetus has a serious or unexpected condition, called an 'anomaly'.

If this happens, you may be offered a termination to end the pregnancy.

You can speak to the screening midwife to learn more about the condition.

Unless you are becoming unwell, you can take time to make your decision.

If you decide to have a termination, you will usually be offered the option to take some medicine to end the pregnancy, or to have surgery to remove the pregnancy.

You can choose if you want to see or hold your baby, and if you would like to have a funeral. There is no 'wrong' or 'right' decision, and the hospital staff can talk to you about your decision.

Understanding what has happened, emotions and mental health

It's very common for people who have a pregnancy loss to ask if they made it happen or could have done something to stop it. As I said before, most times pregnancy loss is not anything that can be prevented, so it isn't something you could have changed. But this doesn't mean it's easy to understand what happened to you.

Having an answer as to why this happened can be comforting, but very often health professionals do not know why a person has a pregnancy loss.

Finding a way to process your grief can help with this uncertainty. You might want to search online for 'pregnancy loss charity' and the name of your country to find local sources of support.

You may find that helplines or social media for pregnancy loss can help you to feel less alone. Being Autistic, you may find that your experiences and feelings are different to some of the non-Autistic parents. If these spaces are not helpful for you, do not feel that you have to use them.

You and your partner may be able to support each other through the loss, but it can be common for couples to struggle to talk about pregnancy loss together, despite their shared grief.

Counselling can help give you the space to think through your emotions. If that isn't available to you, you may find that journalling is a way of processing some of your grief and thoughts.

Overall, it's really important to be kind to yourself at this time. If you need to take time off work, that is absolutely OK.

If you are feeling very depressed, are drawn to self-harm, or are having thoughts of suicide, it is time to get professional help.

! Be very kind to yourself after pregnancy loss. Try to find a way to process your thoughts and feelings, but keep in mind that this was not your fault.

Pregnancy after a pregnancy loss

If you have experienced a pregnancy loss, you are slightly more likely to experience another pregnancy loss in the future. With miscarriage, the risk of having another miscarriage slightly increases each time you have a miscarriage.

It may be that you and your partner decide to try to get pregnant again as soon as possible, or you may decide that you need to wait to process the loss.

If you want to try again, there is no medical reason that you need to wait to try. If you are having tests to find out why you had a loss, it might be helpful to have them first.

Some people will decide that they cannot cope with another loss, and will decide not to get pregnant in the future. There is no wrong or right decision, and each person must do what feels right for them.

We do know that in a general group of people who have experienced pregnancy loss, it is normal to feel worried and anxious about losing another baby.

What Autistic people said... about their pregnancy after loss experience

- Most people felt really anxious about the possibility they would have another loss.
- Some people really wanted to have a child, but felt too anxious to continue trying to conceive.
- For those who had another pregnancy, it could be very worrying the whole way through the pregnancy; some people became hyperaware of small changes to their body.
- Some people felt intense grief or feelings of loss for the pregnancy (or pregnancies) they had lost during their following pregnancy.
- Some wanted to be happy during their pregnancy, even if they knew they had a higher risk of a pregnancy loss.
- Talking to people with similar experiences could help.
- Letting midwives know they'd had a previous loss could mean they were more sensitive.

Conclusion

You've made it to the end of Chapter 6! We've covered lots of different things related to pregnancy complications and the tests and treatments you might be offered if you experience them. We've also thought about pregnancy loss: something that happens in around one in every four pregnancies. As always, if you are worried about bleeding, changes in movements or anything else, please do contact your local maternity unit straight away, day or night. If you have experienced a pregnancy loss, I'm very sorry for your loss. Please be very kind and gentle to yourself. There is no need to rush into trying to get pregnant again if it feels too soon. In the next chapter we'll be thinking about changes to your body during pregnancy, including sensory changes and the changes that happen to most people in late pregnancy, although it's OK for you to go to whatever section you like.

CHAPTER 7

Changes to Your Body and Mind Shortly Before Birth

CONTENTS

Introduction

This chapter aims to make sure you know what to expect from your body late in pregnancy.

First, we think about relationships and setting boundaries. This includes a tool to help you identify your boundaries about how you and the baby are treated after birth.

Second, there will be quite a lot of changes to your breasts, including producing 'colostrum', a type of very concentrated milk ideal for newborn babies, in the third trimester. We also think about buying pregnancy and nursing bras.

Third, we think about changes to your genitals as they get ready for you to give birth. This includes things you can do to reduce the likelihood of a 'tear' during birth. Another thing that happens to some people after they give birth is peeing when they don't want to, such as when they laugh or cough ('stress incontinence'). Exercising your pelvic floor muscles during pregnancy can reduce the chance of having stress incontinence after birth. It can be harder for Autistic people to find their pelvic floor muscles, so we talk about this.

Lastly, we focus on the changes related to your genitals. First would usually be a 'show' or a 'bloody show', which is when the mucus plug that has blocked your cervix comes away into your underwear, sometimes with a small amount of blood. Second, we'll think about your waters breaking. Finally, we'll think about contractions; sometimes these are you going into labour, but other times they are a false alarm, known as Braxton Hicks contractions.

Relationships and finding your boundaries

In Chapter 2, we talked about how many Autistic people have worse sensory issues during pregnancy. If it's been a while since you looked at that chapter, you might like to have a look now. The key message is to allow yourself to stim and do activities that help you to self-regulate.

Later in pregnancy, this is still really important, as being under stress when going into labour can result in more complications. By complications I mean your labour slowing down or stopping, or needing help to get the baby out using forceps or a caesarean section. These can be really hard on you and baby.

Relationships

Relationships in pregnancy

Relationships with your partner and family can change during pregnancy, and after birth.

One thing that can be helpful to discuss with your partner is what you each do that makes the other one feel loved. By knowing this, it means you have a better chance of keeping that 'love language' going after birth.

It is safe to have sex (and orgasms) in pregnancy, unless your midwife has told you not to. But many people find that they want less sex when they are pregnant. This can be because some positions put pressure on your bump and are uncomfortable. You may also find your breasts are more sensitive and can be painful if touched.

If you have bleeding during pregnancy, including after sex, you should get checked by your health professional. If you have been bleeding, leaking fluid from your vagina, or your midwife is worried about your cervix, you may be told not to have sex.

One thing that you shouldn't feel pressured into during pregnancy and after birth is sex, even if your partner tells you that is the only way they feel loved by you.

Some parents who are in a relationship take a 'babymoon' in the second or third trimester of pregnancy, to have time to bond before baby is born.

What is a babymoon during pregnancy?

There are two types of babymoons – before and after birth.

Here we're going to talk about a babymoon before baby is born.

Babymoons are times for the family to bond, like a honeymoon is to help a couple bond after their wedding.

During pregnancy this means some uninterrupted time for you and your partner to feel emotionally connected to each other and loved.

Many people go away for a babymoon, but if you're on a budget it could be as simple as having an uninterrupted weekend together at home where you only do things together that you enjoy.

The idea is that this time sets you up to be united and a strong family unit when baby joins you.

Preparing for good relationships after birth

Thinking about the time after you've given birth, if people around you are doing things you find stressful, your energy is more likely to be stretched thinly, which might lead to shutdowns, meltdowns and longer-term Autistic burnout or postnatal depression (see Chapter 13 for more information).

So, it might be helpful if you can identify things that cause you stress or take up a lot of energy, and try to find solutions. The tools in Chapter 2 give you some ideas focused on the sensory world (see page 31), and things that help to reduce your stress or overwhelm (see page 34).

You could think about stocking up your freezer with safe foods or meals you've frozen. This will save energy after birth.

Another thing that can cause you stress is interactions with people. There are some ideas in Chapter 2 (page 33) on how you can ask people to stop doing things you find difficult.

In addition, now that you are closer to birth, it is more important to think about the rules or boundaries you would like for how people interact with you and your baby during and after birth. Boundaries are the way that you tell people how they can respect your needs.

These needs can be physical, like making sure you get enough rest, that you are able to eat and drink regularly, that you have time with someone else looking after the baby to help you re-regulate, or that you get to hold the baby as much as needed to breastfeed. We also have emotional boundaries, which can include having enough privacy, support and social connection.

Being Autistic, you may feel that you routinely put your needs and comfort aside, so that other people get their needs met. However, having a new baby is a major life event, and these boundaries can be important in keeping you well, which also helps you to meet your baby's needs.

Some people decide to give a vague ('baby's due in March') or false (later) 'due date' to those they think might be difficult to manage. This means that when the time comes for you to give birth, you won't have the pressure of people knowing.

There are no right or wrong boundaries, it's whatever makes you (and your partner, if relevant) comfortable.

You can watch an Autistic antenatal educator talk about changing relationships in pregnancy here:

Tool: Thinking about your post-birth boundaries

Boundaries are unique to you, but these questions might help you think about what would ideally happen to you around birth and the fourth trimester:

- **Support:** Would you like somebody to be with you during birth? If so, who? How can they best support you (we will talk more about this in Chapter 8).
- **Support:** Are there any things you definitely don't want someone to do during birth?
- **Privacy:** Would you like visitors when you are in hospital? If so, who?
- **Privacy:** Is there anyone you think might turn up at the hospital uninvited? If so, who? How can they be stopped from doing this?
- **Getting your physical needs met:** What are the things it would be helpful for you to have help with after baby is born? For example, cooking meals for you, coming over to do laundry and cleaning, sitting with you whilst you're feeding baby so you don't feel alone.

- **Getting your physical needs met:** What are the things you don't want people to do when they see you or visit after baby is born? For example, touching you, hugging you, kissing the baby, holding the baby, giving advice on parenting.
- **Getting your physical and emotional needs met:** When do you think you might feel OK for people to visit you at home?

Thinking about your boundaries whilst you're still pregnant gives you some time to tell people about your boundaries and for them to get used to them. One thing you could decide in advance is that you will not have visitors after birth for a set time, like two weeks.

If you decide to do this, you could put an announcement up on social media (and even your front door if you think people might just turn up!). It could say something like 'Baby (name) has been born; we are all well. Thank you all for your support and well wishes. We are not having any visitors for two weeks until (say the day and date, e.g. Sunday the 16th).'

What Autistic people said... about boundaries with others when you have a new baby

- Some people meant well, but were unhelpful – like:
  - Offering to cook but making food they didn't like.
  - Only wanting to hold the baby. This meant not doing any useful tasks and making it harder for the parents to bond with baby.
  - It could be hard to say no to help when someone was already doing it.
- Some people had a lot of support from a particular person (often a mother or sister), and found it really valuable. Sometimes other relatives (including mothers-in-law) didn't like that they didn't get the same amount of time with the baby, and it could feel painful enforcing that boundary.

- If they had a caesarean section (particularly if it was unplanned), they might need a lot of help in the first few months as their incision healed.

To help people understand your needs and stick to your boundaries, you are going to have to tell them, even if it is awkward for you. It's important that your words are **clear and direct**, so they understand what you mean.

To make it easier, you could send your boundaries as messages, rather than having a conversation in person or on the phone.

Script: How to tell people your boundaries

You might want to use or adapt some of these phrases:

- 'I would prefer to talk about my boundaries in writing, so there are no misunderstandings.'
- 'I love you, but to stay well after I give birth, I'm going to need to make sure I prioritize my own needs.'
- 'I do not want anybody to visit the hospital when I am having the baby. It would make me stressed and worried and that can have negative impacts on labour.'
- 'After I've given birth, it would be really helpful if you could (do thing), but we have decided that we don't want people to (do other thing). Is that OK with you? If not, we won't be able to see you until (later time).'
- '(partner) and I have decided that we are not going to have visitors for the first month after baby has arrived. This is to give us time to bond as a family.'
- 'After baby has been born, I don't want anybody to kiss them. This is because it can pass on colds and other illnesses that can make babies very poorly.'
- 'We have decided (boundary). Please respect our decision.'

Some people will push back against your boundaries, for example family may insist that they should come to the hospital to visit you or come to stay with you after birth.

If you are worried about people trying to come to the hospital whilst you are giving birth, you can tell your midwife or health professional that you don't want any information given out about you, or that information should only be given to specific people, such as: 'I only want my birthing partner, who's name is (say their name), to be given information. Please don't tell anybody else that I am here.' Some hospitals allow you to set a password that people would need to give when they phone to ask about you.

If broken boundaries do not have consequences, the person is likely to keep on breaking your boundary.

Script: How to reinforce broken boundaries

- 'No, we have been clear we do not want you to (do that thing).'
- 'Please stop. You are ignoring the boundaries I told you about.'
- 'You keep on doing things I clearly told you I don't want you to. We need to have a break for a while; I will contact you when I am ready.'
- '(name), I've asked you several times not to (boundary) and you have just done it again. You need to leave my house now, and I will speak to you later.'

Now we've thought about how pregnancy can affect stress and relationships, let's think about how your body changes in the lead-up to birth.

Changes to your breasts

How your breasts change during pregnancy

During pregnancy, your breasts will grow because of the pregnancy hormones, which tell your body to get ready for breastfeeding (even if you don't plan to breastfeed). There isn't a set time when this happens, it can be from around six weeks to six months. Many people find that their breasts go up one or two cup sizes.

As well as this, the brown or pink area around your nipple (the areola) will darken and get more prominent. Your nipples will also get more sensitive and erect.

You may also notice that your ribs have expanded to make space for the baby as it grows, meaning you may go up a band size or two.

You can watch an Autistic lactation consultant talk about the changes to breasts during pregnancy here:

Pregnancy and nursing bras

Maternity bras aim to be particularly comfortable during pregnancy, and some can also double up as a nursing bra. The difference between a regular bra and a nursing bra is that the cups of a nursing bra are attached to the shoulder straps by a clip, which can be released to expose the breast whilst still wearing the bra.

Your breasts may grow throughout pregnancy, so you may prefer to buy less expensive bras if your pre-pregnancy bras get too small. You might also want to buy a bra that fits comfortably on the tightest hooks, to allow for additional growth.

If you are planning to breastfeed, you may want to buy some nursing bras in the last few weeks of pregnancy (when your breast size is most likely to have stopped changing). You may find it helpful to get measured in a shop, or to use the A Bra That Fits calculator (www.abrathatfits.org/calculator.php), and the associated Reddit for fitting advice (www.reddit.com/r/ABraThatFits).

Many people are routinely wearing bras that are too small in the cups, so if you were already wearing a bra that was too small in the cups, you may find that whilst your breasts have only grown a bit, you end up wearing a much larger cup size. The Irish Bra Lady (www.instagram.com/theirishbralady) shows examples of well-fitting bras on people of all different sizes, saying which size they are wearing.

It's particularly important that nursing bras fit you properly, as a bra that is too small or too tight can result in blocked milk ducts, which can be painful and lead to an infection (mastitis). It's also best to avoid underwires in your bras.

The 'swoop and scoop' technique makes sure all of your breast tissue is in the cup.

? How do I check if my bra fits?

1. 'Scoop and swoop' (your breasts into your bra):
   - Put on your best-fitting bra.
   - Put your right hand inside the bottom of the left bra cup and 'scoop' your breast tissue from underneath into the cup, then 'swoop' your breast tissue from near your armpit into the cup.
   - Let everything settle and look at yourself in a mirror. Is there any breast tissue sticking out the top of the bra cup, or is it completely flat against your skin?
   - If there's any breast tissue sticking out the top of your bra, it's probably too small.
2. Check the fit – if any of these happen the bra isn't the right size for you:
   - Any breast tissue is not inside the cup, or it pinches your breast tissue (the cup is too small).
   - The band around your chest rises up at the back (the band is too big).
   - The part of the bra between your breasts (the 'gore') doesn't sit flat against your chest wall (the bra isn't the right shape for you).

If you are thinking you may breastfeed, it's a good idea to make sure you have some clothing that allows easy access to your breasts. This doesn't need to be specific 'nursing' clothing, it can be things like shirts or PJs that have buttons at the front. Some 'wrap' style tops and dresses, and dungarees or loose sleeveless dresses can also be pulled to the side. The Facebook group 'Can I breastfeed in it?' is an excellent resource.

Colostrum leakage and harvesting

In the last trimester of pregnancy, your body will start to produce colostrum, which is the first type of breastmilk your body makes. It is very concentrated and contains antibodies. Even when baby is born, colostrum is usually produced in very small amounts, because newborn babies have very tiny stomachs.

It is possible for many people to harvest some colostrum towards the end of pregnancy. If you are diabetic, it is often particularly recommended that you harvest colostrum. However, you should always discuss this with your midwife as it is not advised for everyone.

When is it unsafe to collect colostrum before birth?

- You have had contractions, bleeding from your vagina or a premature rupture of your membranes (your waters have broken early).
- You have stitches in your cervix (sometimes called a cervical suture).
- You have had a premature labour in the past.

If your midwife recommends you express colostrum and you would like to try, you will be given syringes, caps and labels. If you are not sure, you can ask to be given these anyway, and can make a decision later. This is important as the hospital may not allow you to bring in colostrum that isn't stored the way they expect.

You can watch an Autistic lactation consultant talk about colostrum, including collecting colostrum, here:

If you're unsure of anything to do with colostrum, ask your midwife or health professional.

Before you express, you should ensure you have a sterilized container to catch the milk, and a sterilized syringe for storing the milk. We talk more about hand expressing in Chapter 11; never use a breast pump during pregnancy.

You can keep the sterilized container (with a lid on it) in the back of the fridge (at a temperature of 2–4 °C) for up to 24 hours, and add to it when you express, which can be done a few times a day. Then transfer the colostrum from the container to the syringe, label it with the time, date and your name, and put it inside a resealable bag in the freezer, which should be at a temperature below 18 °C.

You will be able to bring your colostrum into hospital when you give birth. Normally they will be able to put it in their fridge or freezer for you, but it's important to ask about this in advance, including asking whether they have a fridge or freezer.

Script: Some questions you might like to ask about harvesting colostrum

- 'Is it safe for me to express my colostrum?'
- 'When should I start expressing colostrum?'
- 'Can you please show me how to express colostrum?'
- 'How should I store my expressed colostrum?'
- 'What do I need to do if I want to bring expressed colostrum to hospital when I give birth?'

What Autistic people said... about changes to their breasts in pregnancy

- Not everybody had a lot of change to their breast size in pregnancy.
- Some people felt that their breasts became 'heavy' when they got bigger.
- When they started to harvest colostrum, some people said their nipples got more sensitive (and more sensitive again when baby started to breastfeed).

- It took a bit of trial and error to find a pregnancy/nursing bra that was comfortable. Some people wore soft bralettes instead.

Changes to your genitals, and how to reduce the risk of tearing during birth

This picture shows the parts of genitals that are relevant to birth.

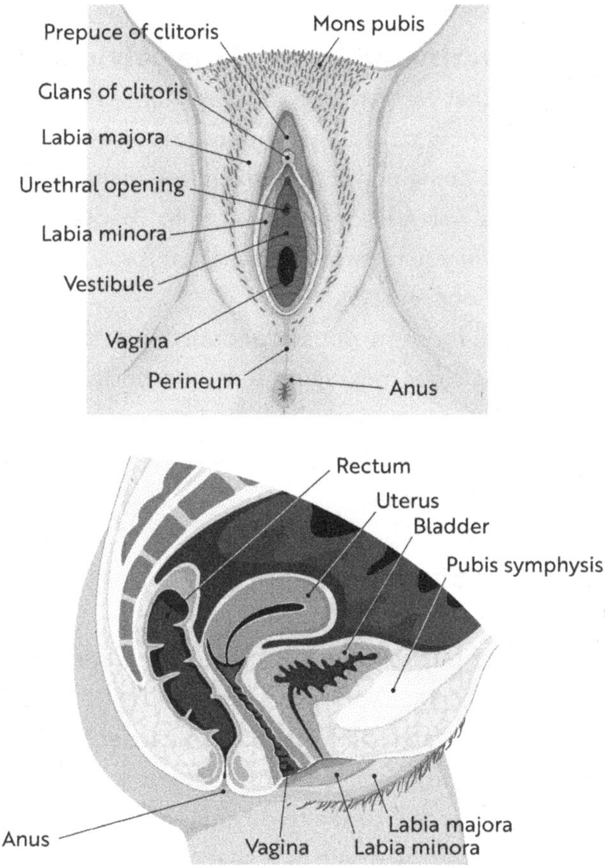

A drawing of internal and external female genitalia

When you speak to your midwife, you can use the language shown in the drawings above, or other words that you are more comfortable using.

When you give birth, your vagina will stretch and change shape to allow the baby's head to come out. But there's another part of your body that also needs to stretch: the perinium.

The perinium is the area between the opening of your vagina and your anus. It includes strong layers of muscles which are part of your pelvic floor. During birth, the more relaxed these muscles are the easier it is for the baby to go down the birth canal. A relaxed pelvic floor also lets the area between your vagina and anus (the perinium) stretch, reducing the chance of a 'tear'.

Relaxing your perineum (part of the pelvic floor)

There are two ways that you can help your perinium get ready for birth: the first is learning how to relax your pelvic floor. We talked about the pelvic floor and doing pelvic floor exercises, including showing a picture of where the pelvic floor muscles are, in Chapter 3 (p. 57), and it might be helpful for you to have a look at that if you aren't sure how to find your pelvic floor muscles.

It may be difficult for some Autistic people to find their pelvic floor muscles due to less clear messaging from the body about internal processes (this is called 'interoception'). You can ask your midwife for help or a referral to a physio ('physiotherapist') if you're struggling to find your pelvic floor muscles.

? How do I relax my pelvic floor?

- Identify your pelvic floor muscles – these are the muscles that you use to stop yourself from weeing (urinating) or passing gas (farting). This may be harder for Autistic people due to differences in interoception, so don't worry if it takes you a few times to do this.
  - It can help to lie or sit in a space where you are comfortable and won't be disturbed.
  - Aim to keep your leg, buttock and tummy muscles relaxed.
  - Imagine that you need to stop yourself from weeing or passing gas, and squeeze the relevant muscles.

- You're doing it right if you feel a tightening around your anus (bum hole) and/or a tightening or lifting in your vagina.

- When you can identify and squeeze your pelvic floor muscles, it's time to work on how to relax them:
  - Squeeze your pelvic floor muscles, and then try to let go so they are completely relaxed.
  - This should mean that all of the muscles in your lower half are completely relaxed (not tense).
  - Do this several times and repeat this daily until it's easy for you to relax your pelvic floor muscles.

Massaging your perineum

Second, massaging your perinium from 35 weeks of pregnancy has been shown to result in less tearing during birth and less pain after birth. It can also make the stretching feeling that the perinium does during birth feel familiar, so it doesn't feel as weird when it happens.

If you don't feel able to do this, that's absolutely fine. Also, if the massage is uncomfortable for you, be very gentle and build it up slowly.

How do I prepare my perinium for birth?

Before you start:

- It's usually best to wait until around 35 weeks of pregnancy; check with your midwife if you want to start earlier than this.
- You should not stretch your perinium without asking your midwife first if you have:
  - genital herpes
  - a vaginal infection like thrush or
  - your waters have broken.
- If your nails are long or pointed in shape, you might want to trim your nails first to avoid injuring your vagina.

- You'll need some plain unscented oil, like olive oil (that you use for cooking) or grapeseed oil, or a water-soluble lubricant like KY Jelly.
  - Don't use baby oil, mineral oil or petroleum jelly (Vaseline).
- You may want to have a mirror that you can use to look at your perinium, especially the first few times.
- Ideally, perineal massage should be undertaken three to four times a week for five minutes each time, but any amount of massage is beneficial.

Getting ready:

- You want to be as comfortable as possible before starting, so make sure you have plenty of time and have the environment around you be as calm as possible.
- Most people prefer to warm up the area first, by having a warm bath or shower, or you could hold a warm (never hot – ouch!) wet flannel to the area.
- Empty your bladder (go for a wee) before starting.
- Wash your hands.
- The exercise involves putting one or both of your thumbs (or your partner's index fingers) into your vagina. Thinking about this, find a comfortable position. You could try:
  - sitting or lying in bed
  - kneeling or being 'on all fours'
  - sitting on the toilet
  - being in the bath or shower, although this may wash the oil away, making it less comfortable.

Doing the massage:

- Put some oil on your fingers and thumbs; you want your vagina to feel well lubricated.
- Start off by putting one or both of your thumbs about five

centimetres (2 inches) into your vagina and resting on the back wall of your vagina (closest to your anus). Let your fingers rest somewhere that's comfortable (on your legs or bum cheeks). If this feels OK, carry on to the next step. If not, get used to relaxing whilst you do this.

- Gently press down with your thumb or thumbs towards your rectum (sometimes called a back passage); stay like this for a minute or two, trying to stay relaxed.
  - You may begin to feel a slight burning or stretching, but it should never be painful.
  - You can use more oil at any point if you feel friction.
  - If your partner is doing the massage for you, it's really important that you can let them know if the stretching feeling is too much, or if it's painful – think in advance about how you can communicate this.
- When you are comfortable with the downward pressure created by both thumbs, you can move your thumbs around the vaginal wall, as though you were making a U shape, trying to keep your pelvic floor muscles relaxed.
  - You should be massaging the inside of the vagina, not just the skin on the outside.
- Once you've done this a few times, you can increase the pressure you use gradually, making sure it's never painful.

Script: Some questions you could ask your midwife about preparing your perinium for birth

- 'I've read about doing pelvic floor muscles to prepare for birth, but I can't find my pelvic floor muscles. Can you help?'
- 'I can't find my pelvic floor muscles. Can you help me?'
- 'I want to try perineal massage. Do you think it's safe for me to start?'
- 'I want to try perineal massage but I have (herpes, thrush, another infection). Do you think it's safe for me?'
- 'I've read about massaging the vagina to stretch it, but I'm

not sure how to do it. Can you show me?' (You should be clear about whether you would like them to show you on a model, describe it to you, or show you on your vagina).

Signs that you're going into labour

When you go into labour, as well as the things that we look at in detail below, you might also feel like you need to do a poo (because your baby's head is pushing on your bowel), or have a pain in your lower back.

If you generally find it hard to sense your body's signals about things like hunger and going to the toilet (you have 'low interoception'), you might not sense your body's signals around early labour. Try not to worry about this, as you will feel the contractions.

In the UK, the guidance from the NHS is to call your midwife or maternity unit **straight away** if:

- your waters break – if they are not clear, you should phone the maternity unit urgently, as baby may have done a poo ('passed meconium')
- you have vaginal bleeding
- your baby is moving less than usual
- you're having three or more contractions every ten minutes
- you're less than 37 weeks pregnant and think you might be in labour.

Also, remember you can phone your local maternity unit any time of day or night if you have any concerns or need some reassurance. This includes if you have any concerns about baby's movements – including moving more, less or changing their pattern.

What Autistic people said... about going into labour

- Some people had 'Braxton Hicks' (practice) contractions the week before giving birth, so knew it was going to happen soon.

- Some had no symptoms until they started getting contractions.
- Some reassured themselves that they were having contractions by putting their hands on their tummy and feeling their tummy muscles tightening and relaxing.
- Timing the gap between contractions was helpful to know that labour was starting.

Mucus plugs and 'bloody shows'

A sign that birth is on the way can be a 'show' or a 'bloody show'. This is when your cervix softens and the mucus plug that has blocked your cervix is released naturally, sometimes with a small amount of blood. If there is more than a small amount of blood, contact your local maternity unit.

This can happen by itself, or can happen if you have a midwife do a 'sweep' of your cervix. We talk more about 'sweeps' in Chapter 8 (page 182).

Not everybody notices when their mucus plug has come away. This is because sometimes you only get a small amount of discharge in your underwear.

The 'show' happens because your cervix is getting ready to give birth. Sometimes when you have a 'show' you may feel cramping, pressure in your pelvis, vagina or back (from the baby's head), or contractions.

There are no hard and fast rules about how quickly you will go into labour after having a 'show', but it's a good idea to let your midwife or doctor know if you think you've had a 'show'.

Waters breaking

Your baby is in a thin bag or sac within the womb. Inside the bag is clear fluid that is sometimes light yellow.

The sac often breaks open during labour, and is sometimes referred to as 'your membranes rupturing'.

In TV shows, when waters break it is often a dramatic gush, with water coming out quickly and contractions and labour happening right away. This isn't always the case.

! On TV, waters breaking looks sudden and dramatic; in real life it's often not like that. Waters breaking can be a trickle over a long time.

For around 9 per cent of pregnancies, the waters break early: before baby is ready to be born (see Chapter 6, page 118, for more information). In other cases, the sac doesn't break, and a midwife or doctor might break it for you in hospital. They use a little thin plastic hook specially designed to do this.

When your waters break, you might feel wetness in your underwear or around your genitals. You might also get a little bit of a leak over quite a long time. For this reason, it can be hard to tell if your waters have broken, or if you have a little bit of pee leaking.

Once your waters have broken, your baby isn't protected by the sac any more and has an increased risk of infection. If you think your waters might have broken, call your local maternity unit. They can give you a physical exam, a scan or both to check if your water has broken.

! If you think your waters have broken, phone your maternity unit; they may ask you to come in to check. This is because baby is at more risk of infection once your waters have broken.

What Autistic people said... about their waters breaking

- The liquid was warm, like pee.
- It could be a small trickle, and feel like if you accidentally pee a bit when you sneeze.
- Some people were surprised at how different it was to how you see it on TV and in films, and weren't sure if it was their water breaking or not.
- For some it felt as though they were peeing, but had no control over it.
- If the waters are broken by a midwife in the hospital, it can feel like a big rush coming out all at once.
- Some people's water didn't break until quite late in labour.

Contractions

A contraction is when your womb muscles tighten, or squeeze, and then release. If you put your hand on your tummy, you can feel your tummy get harder during the contraction, and then relax when the contraction has passed.

There are two types of contractions, and it can be difficult to tell between them.

First, towards the end of pregnancy, your body may have 'practice contractions' where your muscles are getting ready for birth. These are also called 'Braxton Hicks'. Some people feel no pain, but others find them painful (from mild to more severe). They do not usually last very long, and don't get more intense or start to happen with shorter gaps between them.

If you think you might be having 'Braxton Hicks' contractions, but you aren't sure, you can phone your hospital or birthing centre and ask to be checked.

Second are the contractions that are aiming to birth your baby. They can be felt as a tightening in the tummy and sometimes the back and thighs. The contractions soften and open up your cervix and move your baby down the birth canal. This gently opens the birth canal, so baby can be born.

As labour goes on, contractions change in three ways:

- longer – the tightening happens for a longer period
- stronger – the tightening increase in strength
- more frequent – the time between contractions get shorter.

I'm having contractions. When should I phone the maternity unit?

The UK NHS recommend that you phone your midwife or maternity unit:

- if you think you are in labour
- when you are having contractions every five minutes in a regular pattern
- if you're unsure or worried about anything.

Also remember, if you are bleeding from your vagina or your baby is moving less or more or has changed their pattern of movements, it can be a medical emergency – phone your maternity unit straight away.

You can also phone if you need pain relief.

What happens when I phone the maternity unit and say I'm having contractions?

Sometimes the phone is answered by a midwife, but sometimes it's answered by a midwifery support worker or an admin person.

They will ask you some questions. Have your pregnancy notes with you to help you answer.

You might want to tell them that you are Autistic (see Chapter 4, page 73, for script ideas of what to say).

If somebody else phones for you, they might want to hear your answers.

They might also want to listen to how often the contractions are coming, so they can time them.

They will then tell you what they'd like you to do.

This can be:

- phone back if anything changes
- phone back in a set time (e.g. an hour) to tell them how you are
- come in to be checked.

If you are not happy with their advice, you can ask to speak to a midwife or the midwife in charge.

You can also go to the hospital without them telling you to. If you do this, you would then tell them you want to be checked.

There are lots of pain relief options to help you cope with contractions. We talk about this in detail in Chapter 9.

What Autistic people said... about contractions

- People said they felt:
  - similar to their period cramps, bowel cramps or pain from endometriosis
  - completely different to period cramps – more intense, or even 'sharp'
  - like the muscles were pulling
  - that they felt most intense in the middle of a contraction – so it started to build up, peaked and then started to reduce a bit at a time
  - like it was pulsing.
- Talking about the intensity of the pain:
  - Some people didn't feel pain with them initially, just a strange tightening of their tummy muscles.
  - They were **incredibly** painful for many people, especially close to birth.
  - Some people said it was the worst pain they had ever felt.
  - Other people had similar feeling contractions the whole way through.
- They could be felt in the tummy, back and cervix, depending on the person.

This Reddit thread has a lot of Autistic people's experiences of contractions:[1]

This information might make you feel worried, but in Chapter 9, we'll

1 This was available at the time of writing. Sorry if it's been deleted.

talk about pain and all of the different types of pain relief that can be used to manage contractions.

Changes that are not normal and how and when to seek help

In Chapter 6 we talked a lot about signs that something might be wrong with a pregnancy, such as bleeding, pain and baby changing their pattern of movements.

Later in pregnancy this is still very important. There is a short recap below, but please return to Chapter 6 for more information.

If you are bleeding, especially if it is soaking pads or you have pain, it is **very important** to phone your maternity unit for advice.

! Heavy bleeding from the vagina in pregnancy is a medical emergency – please contact your maternity unit for advice.

All babies will have their own unique pattern of movements. You will get to know this throughout the second half of your pregnancy. Your baby should continue moving in their usual pattern right up until the end of your pregnancy. You should also continue to feel them moving when you are giving birth.

! You should continue to feel your baby move all through the third trimester, including when you're giving birth.

It can be normal for all pregnant people to wonder if they should phone the hospital. For Autistic people, we have often had negative experiences in healthcare situations and might find it difficult to get our needs met. Please don't let these bad experiences put you off; bleeding, changes in the pattern of movements or you feeling very unwell can be signs that the baby is not well. Getting medical advice can be lifesaving for your baby.

Maternity units are open day and night. The staff don't mind you phoning up when you are worried. They will ask you some questions, and ask you to come in for a check if they are worried.

An Autistic midwife's top tips... on the days and weeks just before birth
By Diane Fox, RM, PGCPSE PGDPSE

- Always phone the hospital if you have any concerns or need advice or support.
- Make sure you have discussed your needs/wants/desires/ reasonable adjustments with your partner prior to labour. That way they can be your advocate if needed. Write it all down if needed
- Understand the physical changes in your body at each stage of labour so you can visualize the process. Things will happen when the time is right for your body at a pace that is right for you.
- Know the route to the hospital and where to park. Have a practice run, and add in rush hour traffic timings if needed.
- Have a second person you can call in an emergency if needed to drive you to the hospital if your partner is not available.
- Have an emergency person on standby that you can call to drop things to you at the hospital if needed.

Conclusion

You've made it to the end of Chapter 7! We've covered lots of different things related to changes in late pregnancy. First, we thought about managing stress. We then covered changes to your breasts and genitals as you are getting ready to give birth, and thought about things like nursing bras and pelvic floor exercises. We then thought about the changes in your womb (uterus) shortly before birth, including seeing a 'bloody show' in your underwear, contractions and your waters breaking. We then had a recap of signs that you should get checked over at the maternity unit, including bleeding, pain and changes in your baby's movements. In the next chapter we'll be starting to think about birth, including places where people give birth, and inductions if you go beyond your 'expected date of delivery', although it's OK for you to go to whatever section you like.

SECTION II

BIRTH

CHAPTER 8

Birth (1): Where to Give Birth, 'Due Dates' and Inductions

CONTENTS

Introduction

This chapter starts by talking about your right to say no to treatment. This includes some 'scripts' you can use to uphold your rights.

I then talk about the different places you can give birth, like a medical ward in a hospital, a midwifery-led unit or at home. The location has an impact on the pain relief that you can have.

Next, we think about 'due dates', including that they're not the day most babies are born. We talk about what might happen to try to speed up your birth starting. This includes having a 'stretch and sweep' or an 'induction'.

We then start to think about things that might help you during birth. We think about people, the environment around you, moving your body ('stimming') and what to pack to take to the hospital.

At the end of the chapter is the beginning of a birth plan template that you could use. This is based on the things we've spoken about in this chapter. We'll add things to the birth plan template in the next two chapters too. The full birth plan template is available online and can be downloaded at www.jkp.com/catalogue/book/9781839978609

You're allowed to say no to treatment

We talked about this in Chapter 4, but it's so important I'm saying it again here. When you are having any medical treatment, it's really important that you have **informed consent**. This means:

- you understand what the treatment is
- you agree to having it.

The 'informed' part means that the midwives and doctors should tell you what the treatment is, why they think you should have it, and any evidence of risks or benefits that come with the treatment.

You can watch an Autistic antenatal educator talk about the importance of having the information needed to make an 'informed decision' here:

The 'consent' part means that you can say no to the suggested treatment, even if the health professionals think you need it. The only time they can decide to proceed regardless of your decision is if your life or your baby's life is at immediate risk and they decide you can't make the decision (you 'don't have capacity').

You can watch an Autistic psychotherapist talk about your rights during birth here:

Just because you have the right to say no to treatment, it doesn't mean it's always easy to enforce it. Some Autistic parents find communicating with maternity professionals confusing or frustrating.

You can watch an Autistic parent give their tips on communicating with maternity staff here:

If you think this could be difficult for you, especially if you think your birthing partner may struggle too, you could hire a doula (see Chapter 5, page 103) or ask to have an advocate. In the UK, your local council is who you have to ask to get an advocate. It may take a while to organize this, so it's best to start early.

You can say no to any treatment you don't want. If you'd find that hard, look into having an advocate or doula to support you.

Script: Ways to say no to treatment without saying 'No!'

- (if you are being touched, before they have explained the treatment) 'Is this a medical emergency?' (if it is not an emergency) 'Please stop touching me, I'm Autistic and I need to know what you're going to be doing in advance.'
- 'Can you please explain to me why you think I need this treatment?'
- 'What are the risks if I have the treatment? What are the risks if I don't have the treatment?'
- 'I still don't understand, can you please tell me exactly what would happen if you did the treatment?'
- 'Can you please use plain language? I don't understand some of the words you are using.'
- 'Please wait a minute, I am not ready.'
- 'Stop, that's painful.'
- 'Stop, I wasn't expecting you to do that, I need a moment. Can you please tell me exactly what you will be doing, so I don't have any more surprises?'
- If you would find it difficult to say things out loud, you can write them down or use an app on your phone to speak for you (see the section 'But what if I struggle to speak?' in Chapter 3, page 60).

You can watch an Autistic midwife talk about how to ask for support in hospital here:

In many countries, disabled people (including those who are Autistic) are entitled to 'reasonable adjustments' or 'accommodations'.

This includes the way that medical information is provided to you, to make sure that you fully understand the information and that you have enough time to ask questions and process the information.

In some maternity services, you can have a 'flag' put on your maternity notes to say that you need adjustments. Sometimes they might have 'personalized care plans' or 'hospital passports' where information can be added. Sometimes there will be an 'inclusion midwife' or mental health midwife who can help you with this. Ask if there is one in your hospital.

If you are creating a birth plan, you should also include any adjustments you need to process information, as well as anything else to do with the environment and communication. We will talk more about these other kinds of accommodations later in the chapter. At the end of the chapter, there is the beginning of a birth plan which contains information about your preferences and needs for the environment and communication.

You can watch an Autistic parent talk about asking for adjustments (before she knew she was Autistic) in hospital here:

If you need any changes to make the environment around you feel comfortable or to communicate with the staff, you can put this in your birth plan.

For some treatments, like being taken to theatre for a caesarean section, you will be asked to sign a **consent form**. You should always be talked through the procedure first so you understand what will happen, and what the risks are. That said, some birthing people have said that they were asked to sign consent forms without knowing what was on them, because their baby was becoming unwell.

To help prevent this, in your maternity appointments, you can ask questions about what would happen if you needed to have an emergency caesarean section to help you understand the procedure. If you are very worried about this, you could also ask to be shown the forms and discuss any concerns about signing them before you give birth. This would be a disability adjustment to help you decide and agree (give 'informed consent').

What Autistic people said... about being asked to consent to treatment during birth

- Some people said they weren't asked to consent, things were just done. This included vaginal exams (putting fingers into the vagina).
- Some people said they were told 'I'm just going to... (do a thing)' at the same time the person started to do it, so there was no time to say no.
- Some people said that when they said 'yes', they didn't understand what was going to happen, so were surprised (in a bad way).
- Some people found it hard to say 'no' even when they really didn't want the treatment.
- Some people had a birthing partner (often their partner or mum) speak up on their behalf to make sure they got enough time to understand what the health professional wanted to do.

Location

Some people say they'd like to give birth at home, so they'll have more control of the environment. Others would feel more confident in hospital, so there are midwives and doctors available if anything goes wrong.

Either one of these approaches is absolutely fine.

If you give birth at home, once the midwife arrives, they will stay with you once you're in established labour until a few hours after you give birth.

If you give birth elsewhere, the midwife or doctor won't be in the room with you all of the time. They will come in to check you regularly.

You can always ask for help by pressing your call bell, or if it is urgent or you are worried, by sending your birthing partner out to find somebody.

If you give birth at home or in a birthing centre that isn't in or next to a hospital, if anything goes wrong, you will need an ambulance to take you to hospital. You should think about how far away the hospital is and how quickly an ambulance might be able to get to you.

Also, after you've given birth, if you need to go to hospital, in some areas you and the baby will have to go in separate ambulances.

The most relevant thing is that it is better to give birth where you feel comfortable. This is because when you are in labour your body produces the hormone oxytocin, which makes you have contractions. If you are stressed, you may produce less oxytocin, slowing down your labour.

! You get to decide where you want to give birth. The health professionals can only make suggestions.

To help you decide on the best place for you to give birth, you could ask for a tour of the midwifery-led unit and the obstetric ward. You could also ask for a video or photographs of the wards too, with information about where you are likely to be at each stage of birth.

You can also write down questions before your antenatal appointments to ask about what it would be like to give birth in these places.

Below you can see a table which briefly covers:

- each of the places you can give birth
- if a midwife or doctor would be with you
- the type of pain relief available in those places
- what the space might be like
- how much medical intervention you can have.

We will talk about each of these in more detail next.

What types of pain relief and treatment can I get in different birthing locations?

Location	Midwife present?	Doctor present?	Types of pain relief	Environment	Medical intervention
Free birthing at home	No	No	Non-medical only (including TENS machine)	Your own home; full control	None
Home birth	Yes	No	Non-medical (including TENS machine), gas and air	Your own home; full control	Limited
Midwifery-led unit/ birthing centre – not near a hospital	Yes	No	Non-medical, gas and air, midwife-given injections	Aims to be homely and calm; may have birthing rooms with beanbags or pools. Some control over environment.	Sometimes (monitoring baby, 'stretch and sweep' of cervix – see later in the chapter, page 182)
Midwifery-led unit – in or beside a hospital	Yes	Sometimes	(as above)	(as above)	(as above) Can be easily moved to obstetric ward if needed
Obstetric unit	Yes	Yes	All pain relief, including epidurals	More clinical; least control over sensory. Will have a private room during birth. May have a private bathroom.	More likely to happen, but depends on how busy the doctors are.

Giving birth at home

If you give birth in your own home, you get to have much more control over the space around you (the environment). Also, there are fewer medical options available. This could be a good thing, as it reduces the type of interventions you can have. It could also be difficult if any complications happen, or if you decide you would like pain relief that only a doctor can give (including an epidural).

If you plan a home birth, a midwife will visit you at home about three weeks before your due date. They will fill out a form, saying if there are any risks, like if it would be difficult for an ambulance to get to your home.

If you want to have a birthing pool at home, in the UK you need to hire or buy the pool. When the midwife visits, you can ask them about where it would be best to put the pool. This includes things like making sure there is enough space around the pool.

When having a home water birth, it's your job to set up the pool and make sure it's properly clean. You'll also need a thermometer to check the temperature and a sieve to collect your poo. This is because around half of parents do a poo when giving birth, which is completely normal. Ask the midwife if you're not sure about any of this.

This visit is a good time to talk to the midwife about back-up plans for birth in case you need to move to hospital during or after birth.

If you're planning a home birth, your GP can prescribe painkilling injections that the midwife can give you, but this is rare. Ask your midwife during a maternity appointment if you think you would like this.

For most home births, one or two midwives will be with you throughout. However, if you plan a home birth and there aren't enough midwives available that day, they may urge you to come into the hospital instead.

Also, if you have a home birth and the midwife gets worried about you or your baby, they might recommend that you move to hospital. Things they might worry about include labour slowing down or stopping ('not progressing'), baby being 'in distress' (having a lower heart rate), baby not moving much or stopping moving, or you being very tired or bleeding heavily.

Because there is always a risk that a home birth won't happen at home, it's a good idea to pack a bag ready for the hospital before you go into labour. If you need to move to the hospital from a home birth, the midwife will phone an ambulance for you.

Home births might not always be able to happen, so it's a good idea to pack a bag for the hospital. You should pack one bag for you, and another bag for baby.

A second type of home birth is known as **free birthing**. This is where you give birth without any medical professionals being with you. Legally you are allowed to have a free birth, but if you wish to have one, you may face pressure from health professionals because there would not be a medically trained person there if something went wrong.

You can watch an Autistic antenatal educator talk about giving birth at home here:

What Autistic people said... about having a home birth

- Many people made the space around them fit what they wanted, including having a water birth, low light and music.
- Most people had really positive home birth experiences, and said they'd have another one in the future.
- If they'd had a hospital birth before, most people preferred the home birth.
- Many said it was nice after birth to be at home and be able to have peace and rest immediately.
- A small number had to transfer to hospital because they were getting very tired after a long labour.

About why they didn't have a home birth

- Many people were concerned about what would happen if something went wrong.

- Many people were thinking about the reduced pain relief options if they were at home.
- Some people said they knew they would find it too difficult if they needed to go to hospital in an ambulance part way through giving birth.
- Some people said they didn't want anything to go wrong in their home (where they would be reminded of it afterwards).
- Some people had other children or people in their home, so it wouldn't be a space they could control.
- Some people were having a 'high risk' pregnancy, so knew they shouldn't have one.
- Some people outside of the UK wanted one, but couldn't afford it, as it cost more than a hospital birth.

? What do I need to think about if I might want a home birth?

- How far are you from the hospital? This is relevant if a complication did happen, especially if you are free birthing (with no medical support).
- How important is it to you to have:
  - Your birth plan followed – would you feel extremely upset if a midwife wasn't able to come to you when you're in labour?
  - Access to all pain relief options? (See later in the chapter for non-medical and midwife-provided pain relief).
  - Control over your environment? This can include things like you renting a birthing pool, and moving around your house as you wish.
  - Limited medical intervention, such as having your waters broken, continuous monitoring and episiotomy (see page 223).

Midwifery-led care

There are some hospital wards and birthing centres that are run by midwives. These places are often called midwifery-led units or birth centres. If your pregnancy is considered low risk, you will likely be offered the chance to give birth on a midwifery-led unit.

Midwifery-led units can be seen as halfway between a home birth and a birth on a doctor-led (obstetric) ward. The environment may feel less medical than on a doctor-led ward.

Some of these are in a hospital or next to one. Others are not part of a hospital (they are 'stand alone'). Doctors are close by if the midwifery-led unit is in a hospital. This means you have more options for pain relief, as you can transfer to the doctor-led ward if you need an epidural. Help may also be quicker if there is an emergency during birth.

! To have an epidural or doctors helping baby be born, a midwifery-led unit would need to be next to or in a hospital. Otherwise, you'd need to go in an ambulance to the hospital.

You can watch an Autistic midwife talk about midwifery-led birth care here:

What Autistic people said... about giving birth on a midwifery-led unit

- Many people who were too nervous for a home birth chose the midwifery-led unit because they could have more control over the space.
- People who wanted to give birth in a birthing pool often chose a midwife-led birth, as there weren't always pools on doctor-led wards.
- Some people really didn't want doctors to intervene, like having an unnecessary C-section, so chose a midwifery-led ward.

- Some people found their labour slowed down or they'd been pushing until they ran out of energy, and they then needed a C-section.
- Some people were able to leave hospital soon after birth, which they liked.

What do I need to think about if I might want to give birth on a midwifery-led unit?

- If the midwifery-led unit isn't at a hospital with a doctor-led ward, how far away is it to the doctor-led ward? This is in case you need to be transferred if you need help to get baby out.
- How important is it for you to have:
  - access to all pain relief options (epidurals are not available)
  - access to a birthing pool (there may not be as many rooms with pools on a doctor-led ward).

Doctor (obstetrician)-led care

An obstetric ward is run by doctors, with midwives also working there. It is sometimes called 'consultant-led care'. If your pregnancy is considered high risk, you will likely be encouraged to give birth on a hospital ward. You can also choose to give birth here if you are classed as 'low risk'.

On a doctor-led ward, you are more likely to end up having medical interventions.

You can watch an Autistic midwife talk about giving birth on a doctor-led ward here:

What Autistic people said... about giving birth on a doctor-led (obstetric) ward

- Many people were told they were having a 'high risk' pregnancy, so were advised to give birth on a doctor-led ward.
- Some people had previous bad experience giving birth, or were very scared to give birth so chose to have a C-section.
- The sensory environment could be difficult, with bright lights and lots of noise, but some people said they were given the option to dim the lights.

What do I need to think about if I might give birth on a doctor-led ward?

- If any serious complications happen, you will already be in the best place.
- If your midwife or doctor is telling you your pregnancy is 'high risk' they might push strongly for you to birth on the doctor-led ward.
- How important is it for you to have:
  - access to all pain relief options – all options are available on doctor-led wards, but specialist pain doctors (anaesthetists) can be busy, so there may still be a delay if you want an epidural
  - access to a birthing pool – there is often at least one room with a pool, but they may be being used by someone else.

Planned ('elective' or 'scheduled') C-sections

A C-section is also sometimes called a 'caesarean section' or 'caesarean'.

If your health professional agrees that you should have a planned C-section, they will organize a date for you. This may sometimes need to change if there are people who need an emergency C-section.

Rarely, you could go to the hospital for your planned C-section and find that it can't be done on that day. This would be because of more emergencies needing to be in the operating room than expected.

What happens in the week before a planned C-section?

- Health professionals agree to you having a C-section.
- A few days before your C-section, you go to the hospital to:
  - Have the chance to ask any questions or ask for more information if you are worried about anything.
  - Review some paperwork, including a consent form.
  - Have some blood taken for testing.
  - You may be given some medication to take before the C-section; they will tell you when you should take this.
  - You should be given a leaflet with the information written down.
  - You may be told not to eat from the night before your C-section appointment, and to only drink clear liquids (like water) after a specified time.

Script: Some questions you might want to ask about having a C-section

- 'Can you tell me exactly what will happen step by step?'
  - You can then tell them anything that sounds difficult and ask if you could have adjustments to make it easier.
- 'Do I need to stop eating and drinking before the C-section?'
- 'Will I need to take any medication the night before? If so, where do I get it from?'
- 'When I come into the hospital, where will I wait to have my C-section?'
- 'Where will I recover after my C-section?'
- 'How long do you think it will be before I can go home afterwards?'

It is always best to ask about adjustments before the day of your C-section, and then to confirm the adjustments on the day, to make sure they haven't been forgotten. Below you can see some adjustments that Autistic parents have had and that you could ask for.

What adjustments can I ask for during a C-section?

- Your birthing partner could quietly play some music for you on their phone.
- You could ask for the lights that are over your face to be less bright.
- You could ask if it's OK for you to wear noise cancelling headphones or earplugs (these may need to be cleaned before surgery).

What happens on the day of surgery for a C-section?

- You will go to the hospital.
- A health professional will check your 'observations', using a blood pressure cuff on your arm and a little clip on your finger to test your oxygen level and heart rate (see Chapter 6, pages 120–121, where 'observations' are described in more detail).
- A health professional will check on your baby, including their heart rate and their position.
- Usually, you will be given a hospital gown to wear, which is open down the back.
- You may be given some tight stockings to wear, which reduce the risk of blood clots.
- You will be given an ID band to wear around your wrist; if you have allergies you may be given a second band to wear around your wrist. These can't come off without being cut off, so you will wear it the whole time you are in hospital. It needs to be tight enough to not fall off, but you can ask for it to be looser if it's uncomfortable.

- You will be asked to agree to having a cannula.
  - A cannula is a thin tube into the vein. It usually goes into the back of your hand, your wrist, or sometimes the lower arm or inside crease of the elbow.
  - A cannula is used to give you fluids or medication straight into your bloodstream, during or after surgery.

My birthing partner is going to be with me during a C-section – what do they need to know?

- It's normally OK for birthing partners to be in the operating room during a planned C-section.
- Birthing partners should understand their partner's needs and wishes around birth as they may need to help advocate for things. For example, is it important to reduce the brightness of the lights near your face, or is having skin-to-skin contact a priority after birth?
- Birthing partners are normally given clothing similar to doctors and nurses for when they are in the operating room:
  - 'Scrubs', which are trousers and a top.
  - A hat or something to cover their hair.
  - They may be given covers to put over their own shoes.

What Autistic people said... about having a planned C-section

- Some people were told by doctors that there was something wrong with their baby, so that they would need to have an induction or C-section before their due date.
- Some people were worried about needing to have an emergency (unplanned) C-section, so decided to have a planned C-section to have more control.
- Some people had previous bad experiences giving birth.

- Some people were very scared to give birth so chose this as the way where it was most likely everything would happen as expected.

You can watch an Autistic midwife talk about planned C-sections here:

In Chapter 9, we talk about what happens during the C-section. This includes the pain relief you will have (usually an epidural).

Changing birth location

There are two times when you might be asked to change your planned birth location.

This is before you are in labour and when you are in labour. We'll talk about both of these below.

Being pressured to use a different location before you are giving birth

It's your choice where you give birth, unless you are in the very small minority of pregnant people considered to not have the ability to make the decision for yourself (not having 'mental capacity'). This is when you are said to be 'lacking capacity' under the Mental Capacity Act in the UK.

However, if your pregnancy is considered 'high risk' by your midwife or doctor, you may be pressured to give birth in hospital, including on a doctor-led ward, rather than a midwifery-led ward. If you are being pressured to make a decision on the location of your birth, you might want to ask for more information so that you understand everything.

One way of discussing this with your midwife is the BRAIN tool from Liverpool Women's Hospital. BRAIN stands for: Benefits, Risks, Alternatives, Intuition and Nothing.

Script: The BRAIN approach to asking for information about a test or treatment.
Questions you can ask, based on the BRAIN approach, are:

- 'What are the **Benefits** of me having this (pain relief or treatment)?'
- 'What are the **Risks** of me having this (pain relief or treatment)?'
- 'Are there any **Alternatives?**' or 'Is there anything else I could have instead?'
- Ask yourself: 'How do I feel about it? (This is your **Intuition**).'
- 'What happens if I decide to do **Nothing**?' or 'What happens if I decide to wait?'

You can find out more about the BRAIN approach to asking for information here:

Script: Questions you might want to ask if you are being pressured to use a different birth location
You can use the BRAIN approach to asking questions, or use these questions:

- 'What are the risks (to you and to the baby) of giving birth where I would prefer to?'
- 'How much are the risks reduced if I give birth where you want me to?'
- 'Can you give me any written materials or links to videos that discuss these issues, to help me understand this more?'
- 'Can I have another appointment to discuss any questions I still have?'
- 'How much time do I have before you want me to make a decision?'

If you feel that you are not being listened to, or that reasonable adjustments you are asking for are being refused without a good reason, you can complain.

When you are still in the hospital, you can complain to the midwife in charge. You could also ask if there is a midwife trained to support Autistic or neurodivergent people who can help. In the UK you can also contact the Patient Advice and Liaison Service (PALS) to complain, although there is likely to be a delay in any changes to your care.

There will be information on the internet on how to complain by searching for 'maternity complaint' and the name of your hospital.

Being asked to change birth location during birth

If you've decided that you want to give birth at home or in a midwifery-led unit, there is a chance that something will not go to plan during birth. This could be something to do with you or your baby.

If your midwife thinks that things might not be straightforward or safe, they may recommend that you change from your birth plan. They should explain what they are worried about and why they think you should change location.

It's always a good idea to have a 'back-up plan' for if you need to:

- move from home to hospital (in an ambulance)
- move out of a birthing pool to a different room or to allow for a band to go around your tummy for extra monitoring ('continuous monitoring') of you and baby
- move from the midwife ward to a doctor-led ward, so there is more equipment available if needed.

! Things don't always go to plan during birth, so it's always a good idea to think ahead about what might happen if you need to move to a different location during birth.

If this happens, especially if you need to have surgery, like a C-section or to repair a tear that is serious, things might happen very quickly. You might also be asked to sign a form to say that you agree to the surgery.

To help you feel prepared, you can ask your midwife to talk to you about what could happen in late pregnancy.

If you need an emergency C-section, you might be asked to sign a consent form with very little time.

You can watch an Autistic midwife talk about changing locations whilst giving birth here:

You can watch an Autistic parent talk about their experiences of changing locations, from labour ward to theatre, during birth here:

Due dates and trying to start or speed up labour

Only around 5 per cent of babies (that's 1 in 20 babies) are born on their 'due date'. However, hospitals can become very set on these, even when the person knows exactly when they conceived, and know that the due date is wrong.

In some countries, when you approach your due date, your midwife or obstetrician will start to talk about plans to 'induce', or do things to start, labour.

Once you have gone beyond 40 weeks, midwives may talk to you about things to get your labour started if your birth hasn't started by 41 weeks. This is because the placenta stops working as well. Also, after 41 weeks there is a higher risk of stillbirth or problems for the baby.

The things they offer are medicines or techniques like 'sweeps' and 'breaking your waters'; I describe these below. You can also ask for a copy of your hospital's information on 'induction of labour' for more details.

You can choose if you want to try one, some or all of these. Also, your decision about whether to try these can change over time. For example, you could say that you don't want to try something yet, but you might want to try it in a few days.

You never need to say yes, unless there is an immediate danger to your life or the life of your baby. If you don't want to try to speed up labour, you will be offered extra appointments to check on the baby's health.

If you think that you might find it hard to say 'no', you could write down your thoughts on paper or your phone, or use an app to 'speak' your words for you (see the section 'But what if I struggle to speak?' in Chapter 3, page 60).

> ! You don't need to say 'yes' to things that will speed up your labour unless your health professional thinks there is a risk to you or your baby's life.

You may want to think ahead of time about what would make you want anything to speed up your labour, as you can face **a lot of pressure** from health professionals. This can be overwhelming and hard to say no to. If you are facing pressure to get birth started but feel unsure, you can ask some questions.

Script: Questions you may want to ask when thinking about speeding up labour

- 'Why do you want to do this?'
- 'Is my baby currently showing any signs of distress?'
- 'Do you have any concerns about my health if we wait for natural labour?'
- 'What are the risks of this procedure?'
- 'Is this more likely to make me need a C-section?'
- 'Can you please write down the name of the thing you are suggesting so I can read about it and give you an answer next time?'

You can also use the BRAIN tool to think about your decision (see earlier in the chapter, page 177).

You can ask for a second opinion from another doctor; they might also advise an induction.

Trying to speed up labour naturally

There are natural ways that can help bring labour on, and you may want to suggest trying some of these first if you do not want to try a medical intervention.

How can I get labour to start naturally?

The UK NHS has a number of suggestions.

The most evidence is for using:

- gentle exercise, like walking or bouncing on a yoga ball.

There is some evidence that these natural ways can help:

- acupuncture
- eating dates in the last few weeks of pregnancy
- gently rubbing or rolling your nipples ('nipple stimulation'), because it causes oxytocin to release.

There is no evidence that these ideas work:

- having a spicy curry
- having sex (you shouldn't have sex if your waters have already broken)
- hot baths.

These ideas to bring on labour could **harm** you and **should be completely avoided**:

- castor oil
- evening primrose oil
- clary sage oil.

Stretch and sweeps

Your midwife may offer you a 'sweeps' or a 'stretch and sweeps'.

What is a 'sweep' or a 'stretch and sweep'?

A sweep involves a health professional putting their lubricated and gloved finger into your vagina and then into your cervix, and gently but firmly running their finger around your cervix. The purpose of this is to separate the membranes of the bag of water around your baby (the amniotic sac) from your cervix. Doing this releases hormones which may start your labour.

Some people feel worried about having a sweep, but if you choose to have one, try to be as relaxed as you can. Having a sweep can feel like a lot of pressure on your cervix, and be uncomfortable or painful during and just after the sweep. It can make you have some cramping or a small amount of bleeding. Some people say it feels like a smear test (cervical exam).

If your cervix isn't ready (open enough) for a 'sweep', they can try to stretch your cervix. If they do this, they may offer you another sweep at your next appointment.

Having a sweep increases the chance that you will naturally go into labour in the next two days, especially if your cervix is already getting ready for birth by softening. So sometimes it helps, but it doesn't work for everybody.

You do not have to agree to having a sweep. Also, if you say yes and then change your mind, you can tell them. You can also ask them to stop at any time.

You can watch an Autistic midwife talk about vaginal exams and stretch and sweep here:

What Autistic people said... about having a 'stretch and sweep' or a 'sweep'

- Some people had a lot of pressure from health professionals to have a stretch and sweep.
- Some people found it painful.
- Some people felt that having a 'sweep' didn't make their labour start faster.
- A small number of people had this done without their permission, during a check of their cervix. Understandably, this was very upsetting.

Induction of labour ('being induced')

There are a few different options for doing an induction. These are medicines, a device in your cervix and breaking your waters.

Taking medicine to open your cervix

You can take hormones that can help start your labour. This is usually the first option, which can help your cervix to open.

You can have tablets that you put inside your vagina (a pessary) or a gel that goes into your vagina.

You can also be given tablets to swallow (oral tablets).

If you take this medicine, you will usually stay in the maternity unit.

Cervical balloon

A balloon induction is when a soft tube (catheter) is gently inserted into your womb. Sometimes they will use a speculum to gently open the vagina. This is the same tool used during a smear test (cervical exam).

It can be uncomfortable and sometimes painful to have the tube put in. You can have gas and air for pain relief when they do this (see Chapter 9, page 217).

The tube has a balloon at the top, and some liquid (sterile saline) is put into the balloon.

The balloon puts gentle pressure on your cervix, which might help it to open. It usually stays in place for 24 hours.

You might be able to go home with a cervical balloon in place. You would go back the next day to have it taken out.

If the balloon falls out, you have bleeding or contractions, your waters break or you feel unwell, you should phone your local maternity unit. You will be invited to go in for a check.

'Breaking your waters'

When your cervix is open, if you haven't started having regular contractions, 'breaking your waters' may be offered. This is another way to try to speed up labour.

What is 'breaking your waters' (also known as artificial rupture of the membranes (ARM) or amniotomy)?

If your cervix is open but labour hasn't started, you may be asked to have your 'waters broken' by a midwife.

To break your waters, the midwife uses a small hook to make a tear in the bag of water (the amniotic sac) around your baby.

Having your waters broken may:

- Make your labour speed up, but it doesn't mean that labour will be shorter.
- Make your contractions feel more painful as your body's naturally produced oxytocin hasn't yet caught up with the stage of labour. To help, you might be offered some oxytocin.
- Mean you and your baby are more likely to be monitored than in naturally started labour. This can mean you can't move around as much.

Being given oxytocin

Oxytocin is a hormone that your body naturally makes during labour.

You may be offered oxytocin if:

- Your cervix is open but you are not having regular contractions.
- Your labour isn't going as quickly as expected.
- You have your waters broken (to speed up your contractions).

This would be a synthetic form of oxytocin, which would be given as an IV drip.

? What happens if I'm given oxytocin?

If you are given oxytocin, contractions may start within half an hour (30 minutes), but each person is different.

It is usually given into a tube (cannula) in the back of your hand (see earlier in the chapter for a description of having a cannula).

If it isn't an emergency, you may be able to have numbing cream before they do the cannula. It takes about 30 minutes for numbing cream to work.

You may need to have more monitoring. You can ask if this would mean you need to stay still, or if you would still be able to move around.

Who should be in the room?

Many birthing people choose to have at least one person with them during birth. You may be allowed more than one person to be with you, but you will need to check this with your hospital.

Choosing who should be with you is a very personal and important choice. Ideally, you want someone who you know is going to be able to support you well, which means being able to understand your needs and advocate for you if necessary.

If you plan to let your birthing partner speak for you, sometimes you might be asked to sign paperwork to say that they can give consent (agree to treatment) for you.

You may also want a doula to be present (see Chapter 5, page 103 for more information).

At least as important is who you definitely do not want in the room when you give birth. This can include family members who you would not want present. I say this because social media is full of stories of mother-in-laws and other family members assuming they would be invited and insisting they should be allowed to watch when the pregnant person says no!

You might also want to choose if you want student midwives or student doctors to be in the room; it's your choice.

What sensory environment do you need to give birth comfortably?

If you give birth at home, you have almost full control over the space around you.

If you are giving birth outside of the home, you might want to think about the sensory tools in Chapter 2 (pages 32 and 34), to think about what could be difficult for you and what could be improved.

The standard environment in a hospital can be quite bright and clinical. You might find it useful to take some sunglasses with you.

You might also be able to hear other people giving birth. As well as this, you might hear the sound of alarms going off and machines beeping. You might find it helpful to take earplugs or noise cancelling headphones to hospital. Another option is headphones to listen to music, books or hypnobirthing content (see Chapter 9, page 215).

During birth you are likely to have health professionals ask to touch you. This can include things we talk about more in Chapter 9, like examinations of your bump to check baby's position, putting monitoring on your bump to listen to baby's heartbeat, and vaginal exams. They may also offer massage and help with sanitary pads if needed. Some health professionals will also touch you on the arm or shoulder to try to be reassuring. You can ask them not to do these things, or to always ask permission before they touch you.

In hospital, the temperature is often quite hot, to help babies stay at the right temperature. There may be fans available, but not always. These fans can also be noisy! It might help you to find a small handheld fan, cooling spray or water in a spray bottle that you can take with you. To give birth, you might want to wear a bikini, lightweight dress or nightdress.

Many people also find the smell of hospitals to be unpleasant. You could take along some perfume or lip balm that you like the smell of, to give you something nice to smell.

You can watch an Autistic occupational therapist talk about the sensory side of maternity care and birthing in hospital here:

If you're giving birth in hospital, you might like to pack things to make the place more comfortable, like sunglasses, noise cancelling headphones, a handheld fan, lightweight clothes and perfume.

You can watch an Autistic parent talk about being very sensitive to the things around them, including during and after birth, here:

Some hospitals will give you the opportunity to visit the ward you will give birth on. This is sometimes as part of antenatal classes. Other times they may have a video online that you can watch.

I would recommend visiting or watching the video if you can, as there may be some things that could be easily changed. You can discuss these with your midwife in your antenatal appointments.

How do you communicate pain?

Autistic people tend not to show our pain through facial expressions and noises as much as non-Autistic people. Instead, many Autistic people tend to describe their pain clearly using words.

A common issue in my research has been health professionals not understanding Autistic people's pain presentations. This has included people who were literally about to deliver their baby not being believed that they were in labour.

It may be helpful to think about how you show and communicate about pain. You could write this down on your birth plan.

! Autistic people tend to show their pain less; this means some health professionals don't believe our pain. You can write how you show pain on your birth plan.

'Stimming' during birth

'Stimming' is doing a soothing repetitive movement, like rocking, moving your hands in a certain way or watching something you enjoy. Some parts of stimming can fit with 'hypnobirthing', which we talk about in Chapter 9 (page 215).

Stimming can help Autistic people to stay calm or cope in difficult circumstances (like giving birth!). It's absolutely OK to 'stim' during birth.

You might need to think of what stims you can do if you have to stay still to have continuous monitoring. For this, movement involving just your hands might help the monitor to stay in place.

What should I take to the hospital?

This can be quite individual, but the things listed below might be useful. You can also find lists online, with quantities, if you search for 'hospital bag'.

Tool: Hospital bag packing list

You don't have to take everything on this list.

Things most people need for themselves:

- Maternity notes
- Birth plan
- Loose clothes to wear during labour
- Hair ties if you have long hair
- Lip balm (your lips can get dry with gas and air)

- Dressing gown and slippers
- Nightwear to wear after labour – if you plan to breastfeed, think about easy access
- Comfortable clothes (a few changes in case of bleeding or baby being sick)
- Underwear (knickers rather than thongs, to be able to fit in large maternity pads) – you may want disposable or old underwear as they may get bloodstained
- Maternity pads or super-absorbent period pads (2 packs of these)
- Bras that fit you well – you may need a few as you may leak milk on them – if you plan to breastfeed you may want breastfeeding bras
- Breast pads, to catch any leaking milk
- A spare bag for dirty washing
- Toiletries, including spare contact lenses if you wear them
- Any medicine you take
- Snacks and drinks (if you find eating hard, you may want lots of your favourite snack in case you have to stay in hospital for a few days)

Things to help you pass the time:

- Phone and phone charger (you may need a long charging cable or battery pack)
- Download favourite shows onto a tablet or your phone (the wifi may be bad)
- Music, books, magazines and anything else that helps you to calmly pass the time

Sensory items:

- Sunglasses or an eye mask for bright lights
- Noise cancelling headphones or earplugs to reduce noise, music, audiobooks or hypnobirthing content to listen to

- Battery-operated fan and/or water spray in case it's too hot
- Perfume, lip balm or aromatherapy oils to have something pleasant to smell
- Your own pillow if you are particular (they may not have lots of pillows available in hospital)
- Birthing ball (also called a yoga ball) if you want one and they don't have them
- Things that are nice to touch or hold, like stim toys or soft toys (plushies)
- TENS machine for pain relief (you can hire these) (see Chapter 9, page 216)

Things for baby:

- Clothes, including all-in-one suits and warm clothes if needed for going home
- Anti-scratch mittens and socks
- A hat
- Nappies (lots!)
- Cotton wool pads (like you'd use to take off makeup) or wipes for changing nappies
- A blanket or shawl
- If you plan to formula feed, you may need to bring formula, bottles and teats (see Chapter 11, page 286 to help you choose)
- Muslins (for after feeding)
- A car seat if you're taking baby home in a car

Things for your birthing partner:

- Swimwear if they'll be getting in the pool with you
- Change for the car park (if needed)
- Clothes, phone, toiletries, snacks, etc.

Even if you pack lots of stuff, you may still find you've forgotten something you really want. It's always helpful to have someone on standby who can bring you things you need.

You can watch an Autistic parent talk about sensory care items to take in your hospital bag here:

Birth plan – part 1

In this chapter and the next two chapters, we'll end by thinking about things you might want to add to your birth plan. This means by the end of Chapter 10 you will have read everything you need to think about your birth plan. A downloadable version of the birth plan for you to fill out yourself can be found at www.jkp.com/catalogue/book/9781839978609, as indicated by a ★ symbol.

What is a birth plan?

A birth plan is a document that describes your wishes for birth. It is a record of things like:

- what you absolutely do not want to happen
- what you would like to happen, if possible.

A birth plan can be useful if you're not always able to speak or you can find it hard to say no.

You can watch an Autistic parent talk about their experience of making and using a birth plan here:

You can watch an Autistic midwife talk about things to consider putting in your birth plan here:

Even if you know exactly what kind of birth you want, you might include a 'back-up plan' in case things need to change. So, if you want a vaginal birth, you may still have information about what you would like to happen if you need to have a C-section.

You can watch an Autistic antenatal educator talk about having a back-up plan for your birth plan here:

Do I have to have a birth plan?

No, it's your choice.

Some people don't want a birth plan because it might not be possible to do what it says.

Having a birth plan that has been discussed and shown to your midwife before you give birth may help you to have the environment changed and your wishes followed.

Your birthing partner, or doula if you are having one, can play an important role in advocating for your needs here. Let them know the things that are really important to you, so they can push for these to be included if it would be possible and safe.

Some people use a lot of detail, whilst others keep it quite simple. It's completely up to you.

You can watch an Autistic parent talk about the things they wish they had when giving birth here:

Tool: Birth plan part 1 – where and when to give birth

This is only part of the whole birth plan, and covers the things talked about in this chapter. The full birth plan template with space to write your answers is available online and can be downloaded at www.jkp.com/catalogue/book/9781839978609

Decision to be made	Choices
Location and who should be there	
I want to give birth	At home
	At home – alone (free birthing without a midwife) if necessary
	In the midwifery-led unit or birthing centre – not at a hospital
	In a midwifery-led unit at a hospital
	On an obstetric ward (with doctors present)
	In a birthing pool
	Having a planned (elective) caesarean section
At my birth, I want these people to be present	Birthing partner (name, relationship to me)
	Second birthing partner (name, relationship to me)
	Other, e.g. my doula (name and contact details)
At my birth, I definitely **do not** want these people to be present...	
Staff	I want as few staff as is safe
	I don't want any extra staff, like support workers, cleaners and people serving food, to come in without my consent
	Please put a sign on the door saying, 'speak to midwife before entering'
	I don't mind staff coming into the room
Students	Student midwives can be at the birth
	Student doctors can be at the birth
	I don't want students at the birth

cont.

Decision to be made	**Choices**
Things that try to speed up labour (inductions)	
Stretch and sweep	I do not want a stretch and sweep
	I am happy to try a stretch and sweep
Breaking my waters	I don't want you to break my waters
	I am open to breaking my waters being explained to me if medically necessary
	I am happy for you to break my waters
Hormones in the vagina	I don't want hormone gels or tablets (pessaries) in my vagina
	I am happy to have hormone gels or tablets (pessaries) in my vagina
Devices to encourage the cervix to open (balloon catheter or dilator)	I don't want a balloon catheter or dilator to be used
	I am happy to have a balloon catheter or dilator
Oxytocin drip	I don't want oxytocin to speed up labour
	I am happy to have oxytocin
	I would like numbing cream on my skin if possible before putting in the drip
	Please put the drip in my (choose: left or right) hand
To feel relaxed and comfortable when giving birth vaginally I need...	
Sound	The room to be as quiet as possible
	I do not want small talk with my midwife
	I would like to tell my midwife about some things I am interested in
	I have music or videos I want to be played
	Conversations between health professionals should be outside the room when it would be safe
Lighting	The lights to be as dim as possible
	The curtains or blinds to be closed if possible
	The midwife to use a spot light or torch during delivery, if safe

Touch	Hands-off care as much as possible
	Do not touch me without asking me first and checking that I agree ('give informed consent')
Soothing myself through repetitive movements	I may 'stim' by doing...
To feel relaxed and comfortable when having a C-section I need...	
Staff and communication	Please explain to me who is in the operating room
	I do not want any unnecessary people in the room
	I do not want any unnecessary conversation in the room
	I do not want to be spoken to by health professionals unless needed
	I would like health professionals to tell me what's happening throughout
Sound	I'd like my partner to quietly play some music
	I'd like to wear noise cancelling headphones
Light	I'd like the lights over my face to be dimmed if possible
	I'd like to wear sunglasses or an eye mask (like people wear to sleep)
Seeing baby	I want to be shown baby as soon as is safe after birth
	I don't want to see baby until they have been cleaned up
Skin-to-skin	I'd like baby to be placed on my chest for skin-to-skin
	I don't want to do skin-to-skin
	My partner will hold the baby
What I experience	I may show my pain differently to what you expect to see
	Pain can make me begin to 'shut down' – I may not look like I am in pain, as I internalize sensations
	I **can/can not** rate my pain on a scale of 1–10

cont.

Decision to be made	Choices
When I am in pain	
How I communicate	I may be able to clearly and precisely tell you about the pain I am in; please believe me
	I may not be able to speak
	I use an app on my phone or tablet to say things for me
	My birthing partner is allowed to speak for me
	My birthing partner is allowed to make medical decisions for me

An Autistic midwife's top tips... on planning where and when to give birth

By Diane Fox, RM, PGCPSE PGDPSE

- Use the BRAIN tool (see Chapter 8, page 177) to help make decisions about where to give birth.
- Have a core support network inside and outside the hospital. This could include a partner, doula, advocate and/or another support person.
- Use the birth plan to be clear about your sensory needs and reasonable adjustments.
- Use the birth plan to outline your communication needs.
- Tour the hospital prior to delivery. Ask for a one-to-one tour if possible.
- Ask for a care plan to be completed with you and added to your maternity notes and digital maternity record. This can be done by a specialist midwife such as the mental health midwife.
- Ask for support from the hospital learning disability and Autism team if needed. They can support maternity staff on improving the sensory environment.
- You can print the following 'Letter to Healthcare professional' from the Autistic Girls Network website

and give a copy to your midwife to help them understand your Autistic needs and possible reasonable adjustments: https://Autisticgirlsnetwork.org/pregnancy-information-for-health-professionals

Conclusion

You've made it to the end of Chapter 8! We've covered lots of things to do with getting ready for birth. This includes the different places you can give birth, speeding up getting labour started and thinking about what will help you be comfortable when giving birth. Next, we'll be thinking about what happens when you give birth, including the pain relief options. There are some more decisions to be made and it might be helpful for you to think about these in advance, although it's OK for you to go to whatever section you like.

CHAPTER 9

Birth (2): Giving Birth and Pain Relief

CONTENTS

Introduction

In this chapter we carry on thinking about birth. This time we focus on what happens during birth itself.

First, we talk about the different stages of labour, and knowing when to push.

After this, we talk about the ways that you and baby may be monitored during birth.

We then focus on pain and lots of different pain relief strategies for during birth, including natural remedies, and medication given by midwives and doctors.

Last, we think about things that might need to happen to get baby out – like using forceps or a caesarean section.

Stages of birth

There are three stages of labour. Unfortunately, there is no set time limit on when you move from one to another. One thing that we know can help is oxytocin. On the other hand, stress can slow down labour.

What is oxytocin, and how can it help my labour progress?

Oxytocin is a hormone linked with love and feeling connected to others.

It increases during pregnancy and helps you to give birth by making the uterus contract.

You can increase oxytocin by:

- slowing down your breathing
- focusing on something positive – music you like, good food, feeling connected to your partner, nice smells or anything that works for you.

You can watch an Autistic antenatal educator talk about oxytocin during birth here:

Latent stage of labour

This is when your cervix starts to get ready for birth. It does this by softening and starting to open.

You might start to have contractions, but they'll usually be irregular at this stage. We talked about contractions in Chapter 7 (page 151).

Latent labour can go on for hours or days, so try to eat and drink to give yourself energy for later.

What should I do in latent labour?

If your contractions are irregular and far apart, that means you're in latent labour.

- At night, try to sleep or rest.
- During the day, spend time being active and upright to help baby get into the right position. This will help you move into the next stage of labour.

First stage: established labour

This is when your contractions are stronger and more regular. Also, your cervix will have opened to around 3–4 cm in diameter.

I think I'm in established labour – when do I phone the hospital?

The advice from the UK NHS is to phone if:

- your contractions are regular and happening at least every five minutes
- your waters break (this is important as baby is at greater risk of infection after your waters break)
- you need pain relief to cope with the contractions
- you're worried about anything.

You should also remember that you should always phone if baby's pattern of movements changes, like moving less or more, or if you are bleeding.

If you have already had a baby, the first stage of labour may be shorter than your previous births.

If you are struggling to time your contractions, it may be a good idea to ask somebody to do this for you.

If you give birth in a birthing centre or hospital, your midwife or doctor won't always be in the room with you in the first stage of labour. If you need anything, it is always OK to ask. You can use your call bell or send your birthing partner out to find them.

Second stage: fully open cervix

When your cervix is fully open, to 10 cm, you are in the second stage of labour.

Some people have a 'passive' beginning to the second stage. This means that although their cervix is open enough, they aren't ready to start pushing yet.

The 'active' part of the second stage is when baby is visible and the stronger, pushing contractions begin. This can feel like a strong pressure, pushing the baby down towards your birth canal (cervix and vagina).

Not everybody gets the urge to push. If you aren't sure you could ask your midwife to check by doing an internal vaginal examination. They will be able to feel baby's position and let you know if it's time to start pushing.

The second stage of labour ends with birth. It usually lasts for around three hours for people having their first baby, and two hours if you've given birth before.

Knowing when to push

By itself, your cervix being 10 cm dilated isn't a good reason to push. This is because the baby may not be in the right place. If you are pushing at this time you can use a lot of effort and get very tired before the urge comes.

As labour progresses, most people start to feel an urge to push. If you're giving birth without an epidural, this can come with an increase in pain from your contractions.

The urge to push is sometimes called 'bearing down', or it can be described as 'pushing as though you need a poo'. The urge to push is because of the position of baby's head pushing on your pelvic floor muscles as it goes down into the birth canal. When you feel this urge and push in response to it this is known as 'mother-led pushing'.

This is different to pushing when the midwife tells you to, which is known as 'directed pushing'. You can decide if you want the midwife to tell you when to push, or if you want to 'listen' to your body.

! You can ask your midwife or doctor to tell you when to push, based on readings on a monitor or feeling your tummy to know when a contraction is building, **or** tell them not to tell you when to push. It's your choice.

When you push, it might feel good to make noises, like grunts, groans or even to scream. This is similar to when a tennis player serves; they make noise because of the physical exertion. It's completely normal to be noisy when you are pushing.

! It's completely normal to be noisy when you are pushing – try not to feel worried about the noises you are making.

What can I do to be more comfortable when pushing?

- Get into a position that helps your pelvis to be more open, like kneeling, squatting, standing or leaning over a yoga ball.
- Listen to your instincts; if they are telling you to be in a different position, give it a try (your midwife or partner can help you to move if needed).
- Use pain relief – either natural or medical (see later in the chapter for more details).

What Autistic people said... about 'pushing' during labour

People used a variety of pain relief (discussed more later).

Some people:

- found moaning, or focusing on their breathing, helpful to stop them being overwhelmed
- felt on the edge of being overwhelmed
- found it intense, but not unpleasant
- found this stage happened quite quickly.

Occasionally, people:

- pushed until they ran out of energy, or their baby showed signs of distress, and then had emergency C-sections
- stopped being able to talk (had 'situational mutism') because of the pain or intensity.

Third stage: delivering the placenta

This happens after you've given birth. You can be given medication (an injection of synthetic oxytocin, also called Syntometrine or Syntocinon) to make this happen faster than it naturally happens. We'll talk more about this in Chapter 10 (page 240).

We'll now think about what happens during the birth in more detail.

Monitoring you and baby (during first and second stage of labour)

You can say no to any monitoring you do not want during birth.

Some Autistic people found that during birth it got harder to speak. If this happens to you, you can write it down on paper, buy cards with phrases written on them or use your phone. There are apps that you can use on your phone to speak for you (see the section 'But what if I struggle to speak?' in Chapter 3, page 60).

Feeling your tummy

Your midwife may ask to put their hand or hands on your tummy so they can feel your contractions.

Vaginal exams

In the run-up to birth, and during birth, health professionals caring for you are likely to ask to do regular **vaginal exams**. In the UK, these are usually every four hours. You can say no to having these, or can put conditions on, like only if your birthing partner is present.

It might be best to talk to your midwife or doctor early in your labour to make sure they know your wishes.

If you have had negative or abusive sexual experiences and this may impact how you experience vaginal exams, you may want to tell the health professional. That way they can be more mindful and give you extra time. Also, you are always allowed to ask them to stop, even if you said yes to them doing the exam.

Script: Things you can say if you're worried about having a vaginal exam

Here are some things you could say in response to a request. You might want to practise saying some of these:

- 'Are you worried about the baby, or is it a routine vaginal exam?'
- 'I have had some bad sexual experiences and would feel triggered by a vaginal exam, so don't want one.'
- 'I am Autistic and know that a vaginal exam would be very distressing for me, so I don't want one.'
- 'I am worried it might hurt, so I need your assurance that if I ask you to stop, you will remove your fingers immediately.'
- 'You can do it this time, but I don't know if I'll let you do it again.'

Just because you have said yes to one vaginal exam, doesn't mean that you have to say yes to future ones.

There may be times when your health professional is worried about you or your baby, when it becomes important for them to assess your cervix. This is so they know how to help your labour progress. At this point it may be sensible to agree to having the exam, but you can still always say no. The only time this would be ignored would be a true medical emergency, when you or your baby's life is at risk.

What happens during a vaginal exam?

When having a vaginal exam, you are usually asked to lie on your back, but you can be in a different position if it's better for you.

You are asked to open your legs. You may want to be mindful of how much you are extending your hips and knees if you are hypermobile, have Ehlers–Danlos syndrome (EDS) or have had an epidural.

A midwife or doctor will gently wash the area with wet cotton wool or gauze. They will then insert their lubricated fingers (usually two fingers) into your vagina, to touch your cervix and see how open ('dilated') it is.

They will also feel for the texture of your cervix (how soft it is) and its position in your body. This is used as a way of estimating how close you are to giving birth. I say estimating, because even if your cervix isn't very dilated when you have an exam, it can change at different speeds in different people.

The midwife or doctor will then usually tell you 'You are (e.g. 6) centimetres dilated,' and tell you about where baby's head is (how low down) and the position of baby's body.

Having a vaginal exam may feel uncomfortable. They shouldn't usually feel painful, but some people do find them painful. You can ask for pain relief before vaginal exams, and can always tell your midwife or doctor to stop if you are in pain.

Foetal monitoring

Foetal monitoring is when your baby's heart rate is measured during labour. This is so midwives can watch closely for any changes or concerns.

Foetal monitoring is usually done at regular intervals. In the UK, in the first stage of labour, this will be every 15 minutes, and in the second stage after every contraction. Each time they will listen for around one minute. If the health professional has any concerns, they may check more often.

How will my baby's heart rate be checked during birth?
Usually, they will start by checking your pulse (by putting two fingers on your wrist or neck) and your baby's heart rate.

There are a range of different devices to monitor baby's heartbeat:

- A kind of 'ear trumpet' (a Pinard stethoscope) can be placed onto your bump. The health professional will then put their ear at the end of it, quite close to you.

- A handheld doppler, which is a small ultrasound machine, can be placed onto your bump. It is also called a Sonicaid.

- Electronic foetal monitoring uses another type of ultrasound device that is connected to a monitor using wires. It is used to monitor continuously (all of the time). This creates a continuous reading of your baby's heartbeat, called a 'trace' or CTG (which is short for cardiotocography). There are three ways of doing this:
  - **Both on your bump:** Two plastic discs (transducers) are placed on you using two elastic straps (like a belt) around your tummy to keep them securely in place. One measures your baby's heartbeat, the other measures your contractions. It may be hard to get a good reading of baby's heart rate this way. If there are any concerns, you may be offered an alternative.
  - **One on your bump, one on baby's head:** You'll have one plastic disc on your tummy to measure your contractions. The one measuring baby's heartbeat will be a 'foetal scalp electrode'. This is a very small clip that is attached to a very small wire, that's passed through your vagina onto your baby's head (or bum if baby is breech – that is if baby is coming out bum first). It stays on baby's head until they're born. This doesn't harm the baby, but if you have this type of monitoring, they may have a small graze on their head after birth.

  - **One on baby's head and one in your womb:** When you have the tiny clip on baby's head, they can also monitor your contractions by inserting a tube (an intrauterine pressure catheter) through your vagina into your womb.

- Telemetry is similar to electronic foetal monitoring, but doesn't use wires, giving you more freedom to move around. It isn't available in all hospitals.

You can ask the midwife or doctor to explain what they hear to you, or you can ask for reassurance, such as 'Does everything sound OK to you?'

If there are concerns about you or your baby's health, you may be asked to have **continuous foetal monitoring**.

Why would my health professional want to do continuous monitoring?

The reasons include:

- your midwife has listened to the baby's heartbeat and thinks that they may not be coping well with labour
- you have a medical problem, such as diabetes, pre-eclampsia (high blood pressure), an infection or problems with your heart or kidneys
- if you have previously given birth by caesarean section
- factors relating to your pregnancy, such as being more than 42 weeks pregnant, bleeding from your vagina during or before labour, or being pregnant with twins
- factors relating to your baby, such as being small, premature or in the breech position (their bottom will be born before their head)
- medication you have been given, such as being induced with medication to strengthen your contractions, being given heparin treatment (heparin is a medicine that can reduce the risk of blood clots during and after pregnancy),

or if you have had an epidural for pain relief (you will usually have continuous monitoring for at least half an hour after an epidural or epidural top-up).

If you feel very anxious, you can also request continuous monitoring.

How does continuous monitoring impact the parent?

If you have continuous monitoring, it will reduce how much you can move. This is because you are connected to a machine with wires. If you know that you need freedom to move your body to regulate (stimming), this can be difficult.

If your movement makes the device slip out of place, an alarm will go off (often quite loudly) to alert the health professionals.

You will usually not be allowed a water birth or bath if you have monitoring attached.

The elastic straps across your bump may feel uncomfortable, especially if you find the sensory aspects of some clothing difficult.

Research with non-Autistic people has found that continuous monitoring can be reassuring, but it can also be stressful when staff were not able to frequently check the monitor.

Script: Things you might want to say when asked to have continuous foetal monitoring

- 'Why do you want to continuously monitor the baby?'
- 'I'm Autistic and need to be able to move to self-regulate. Is telemetry available instead of a monitor with wires?'
- 'I'm Autistic and will find it very hard to be still. Could you check me manually every few minutes to give me some breaks?'
- 'I'm Autistic and the sound of the alarm is very painful to me. Is there a safe way the volume can be turned down?' (e.g. 'My birthing partner could come to find somebody each time it goes off if needed.')

What happens if baby's heart rate changes?

Usually changes in baby's heart rate are **not** an emergency. Often there will be small things the midwife or doctor will ask you to do, such as changing position to get more oxygen to the baby.

When a baby's heart rate gets too low during labour, it is called bradycardia. It may also be called 'foetal distress' or you could be told 'your baby is in distress'. This can be a medical emergency, with serious complications for baby.

If it is an emergency, baby needs to be delivered as soon as possible, so a caesarean section or the use of forceps or a vacuum device will be required for the safety of you and your baby. We talk about these ways of getting baby out later in the chapter.

! Usually changes in baby's heart rate are not an emergency. If baby's heart rate gets too low, baby will need to be delivered urgently, using forceps or a C-section.

Taking a blood sample from baby ('foetal blood sampling')

If there are worries about baby, the doctors will be deciding if baby needs to be delivered straight away. If they don't have enough information, you may be offered 'foetal blood sampling'.

This is where a very small amount of blood is taken from baby's scalp (or bottom if they're breech). To do this, you would lie back and have your legs up in stirrups (this position is called 'lithotomy').

The blood test results include things like seeing if baby is getting enough oxygen. This helps the doctors decide if baby needs to be born immediately, or if it's safe for you to continue to deliver without extra help.

Pain during labour

Experiences of pain in labour vary for everyone. For Autistic people, they might vary even more.

What Autistic people said... about pain when giving birth

- Many people found it helpful to prepare ahead of time by knowing what happens during labour.
- Some people had pain, but when they told a health professional, they weren't believed because they didn't 'look like' they were in pain.
- Some people said the pain was really different to anything they'd felt before.
- Some people didn't have a lot of pain, so they could be very close to giving birth without warning.
- It could feel strange that their body felt like it was opening up to give birth without them controlling it.
- Several people used hypnobirthing to manage their pain (we talk about hypnobirthing below).
- Some people found retreating into themselves, by closing their eyes and not speaking, helped.

Some Autistic parents chose to give birth without medical pain relief.

You can watch an Autistic person talk about pain during a birth without medication here:

Other Autistic parents will have a different birth experience, including planned and unplanned C-sections.

You can watch an Autistic parent talk about their experience of pain during and after a C-section birth here:

Occasionally the experience of giving birth can be so overwhelming for an Autistic person that they 'shut down', such as not being able to talk.

> You can watch an Autistic parent talk about their experience of shutting down after birth and the impact on their mental health here:

Pain relief during labour

There are many different types of pain relief available. We are going to discuss:

- non-medical methods
- pain relief given by a midwife
- pain relief given by a doctor.

You can choose a combination of things to help you with the pain, and many people who use non-medical options also use some medicine too.

It's really important that you know the risks, benefits and alternatives to the pain relief that you are being offered, so you might want to find out more about the different pain relief available to you, by discussing it with your midwife during antenatal appointments. You can use the BRAIN tool (see Chapter 8, page 177) to think about this.

You can then add this information to your birth plan.

> You can watch an Autistic midwife talk about pain during birth and how to share your own pain experiences with health professionals here:

Non-medical

Using your breathing

Slowing down your breathing, or even just feeling in control of your breathing, is known to increase oxytocin, which can help birth move along. There is a range of different techniques, but you can choose whichever works for you, or even use your own. The key thing is that you feel in control.

Tool: Breathing techniques for labour

- 'Sigh out slowly' or SOS – where you breathe in through your nose and sigh out through your mouth. This is also described as 'breathe in for two (seconds) and out for three (seconds).'
- Take a deep breath before and after each contraction.

Water birth

Being in warm water is known to provide pain relief during birth. This is because it can increase the oxytocin that your body produces. For Autistic people, being in water can also provide sensory feedback, which can soothe you.

Birthing pools are usually set at a temperature of between 36 °C and 38 °C (98–100 °F). You might want to try being in a bath that's that temperature to see if it's a good temperature for you.

When you are in a birthing pool, there is enough space for you to move your body. You could also invite your birthing partner to be in the pool with you. You don't have to do this, and you can also have them support you from outside of the pool.

You can watch an Autistic antenatal educator talk more about water births here:

What Autistic people said... about water births

- Many people really, really liked being in the pool. It could reduce pain and be a positive sensory experience.
- Some people found they didn't like being in the pool.
- One person found it difficult to push in the pool.
- Some people planned a water birth, but ended up needing strong pain relief (epidural) early in labour, which meant they couldn't use the pool.
- Some people wanted a water birth but on the day weren't able to have one because of availability or health professionals' decisions.

You can watch an Autistic parent talk about their positive experience of water birth here:

Massage

Massage is when you or somebody else manipulates the soft tissue in your body, such as rubbing your neck and shoulders or feet. Massage during birth is known to reduce pain and muscle tension. It can also reduce anxiety and stress, and may release oxytocin, which can help your body move towards giving birth.

If you are someone who enjoys touch, you may want to try massage with your birthing partner **before** you are in labour, to give you an idea of what type of massage you might like. If you are someone who doesn't like touch generally, you don't have to try it at all.

What kind of massage might reduce labour pains?

- Slow, repetitive massage that feels comfortable (not massage that makes your muscles tense) – this causes oxytocin to release, which can reduce pain and help labour to progress.

- Firm, deep massage on your lower back – this causes the release of endorphins, which are your body's natural painkillers.
- Gentle, soothing strokes – this can confuse your nervous system, so it doesn't notice the pain so much.

If at any point it starts to feel uncomfortable for you in any way, ask the person massaging you to stop.

! Massage during labour needs to be for your benefit – if you're not enjoying it, tell the person to stop.

Hypnobirthing

Although the name can sound like you're about to be hypnotized, hypnobirthing is not related to hypnotherapy.

What it means is that you train yourself – sometimes by reading how to do it, and other times by listening to recordings or going to classes – to focus on something other than how intense the sensations and feelings around giving birth are.

Sometimes it's suggested that you should visualize being somewhere you really enjoy. This might be difficult if you struggle to visualize things, like many Autistic people do. If that's the case for you, you could bring images or objects with you that bring you a calming feeling.

Other times, short 'scripts' are used in hypnobirthing. They are like affirmations. Some of these may focus on things like feeling safe, well, not in pain and feeling in control. You may find that it's hard for you to focus on something that doesn't feel authentic to you, so it's always OK to modify the script to something that feels true to you.

Some people will listen to a recorded hypnobirthing reading. If you think that would be helpful but don't like the ones you find, you could try recording your own. You could also write key phrases on cards or Post-it notes and bring them with you, keeping them close to you as you give birth, to remind you of those phrases.

You can watch an Autistic antenatal educator talk about hypnobirthing here:

Warm cloths on the perinium

The perineum is the area of skin between the vagina and anus. You may have already been doing perineal massage, but a warm wet cloth applied to the perinium can soothe the pain associated with 'the ring of fire' when you are pushing during labour. This is because the warmth can help the perinium to relax and open. It can also make you less likely to tear during birth.

TENS machine

TENS machines produce a small electric current. They can help with pain in early labour.

They work by giving you feel-good chemicals ('endorphins') and disrupting the body's pain signals.

If you use a TENS machine, you have electrodes taped to your back either side of your spine. Two are roughly where your bra strap would be and the other two are in line with the top of your underwear. They are connected to a small battery-powered machine that you can hold. This means you can control the intensity of the current.

Pain relief midwives are able to give

There are two main types of pain relief that midwives are allowed to give – 'gas and air' and injectable medications.

You can watch an Autistic midwife talk about the sorts of pain relief midwives can give during birth here:

'Gas and air' – Entonox

Entonox, or 'gas and air', is a mix of oxygen and nitrous oxide. It is given to you via a device you hold in your hand with a plastic mouthpiece on the end. The medicine itself comes through a tube connecting to the supply of the medicine.

If you are in hospital, the tube will come out of the wall, but if you're giving birth at home, the midwife brings a canister of Entonox to your home. The tubes are usually long enough that you can use Entonox anywhere in the room you are giving birth in, including if you are in a birthing pool.

You can keep the mouthpiece in your mouth as much as you want, and can control how much of it you breathe in. For example, you can breathe it in when you start having a contraction, and can inhale more deeply when the pain builds up. When you breathe in the Entonox, it will make a noise, which can be louder if you breathe in deeply. Some people also find it helps to bite on the mouthpiece.

Gas and air can help the body to cope by making the pain less intense. It takes around 15 to 20 seconds for the Entonox to work, so if you start breathing it in when you feel a contraction, it should build up to relieve the worst of the pain.

What are the side effects from 'gas and air' (Entonox)?

Entonox can make people feel a bit sick, dizzy or lightheaded but it quickly goes out of your system. If this happens to you, or if you don't like the Entonox for any reason, you can stop using it. Once you've stopped, it shouldn't take long to stop feeling those side effects.

The UK NHS says there are no harmful side effects for babies from using Entonox.

What Autistic people said... about gas and air

- If their pain was extremely bad before getting to use gas and air, it wasn't always enough to get their pain under control, so they used other medicines too.

- Some people found the noise made when breathing in the gas was annoying, or it gave them a feeling of sensory overwhelm.
- Occasionally people wanted to use it, but it wasn't available.
- People found it useful when having stitches after birth (talked about later), but it wasn't always enough by itself.

Injectable drugs: pethidine, Meptid, diamorphine

There are several different types of drug that can be given by midwives when you are giving birth. Different drugs may be offered in different hospitals, so you may want to ask your midwife about this before you give birth.

If you are planning a home birth, you will need your doctor to prescribe these before you give birth, or your midwife won't be able to give them to you.

These injectable drugs are usually given in a syringe into your buttock (bum cheek) or thigh.

In some hospitals, having an injectable medication may impact your freedom in birth, including:

- being asked to have continuous monitoring (discussed above)
- you might not be allowed to use the pool after the injection, because it can make you feel sleepy.

What side effects can you get with injectable pain relief?

Side effects include:

- Making you feel a bit drunk, dizzy, sleepy or confused.
- Making you feel sick, or making you vomit.
- They can cross the placenta and impact baby if you have them too close to giving birth. So, they're usually given before you start pushing so they don't affect baby's breathing. Your midwife will give you advice on the timing and baby's safety.
- They can affect baby's sucking reflex and baby's first feed.

If you are given one of these drugs, you will usually be given something to stop you feeling sick too. If you are still feeling sick, tell your midwife, as they may be able to give you something else.

! If you feel sick when giving birth, tell your midwife, as there are anti-sickness medicines you can safely take.

Pain relief only doctors are able to give: epidurals

Epidurals are given by specialist pain relief doctors called anaesthetists.

They can usually be given once your cervix is at least 4 cm open, but this might vary by hospital. They take around 20–40 minutes to work fully.

This means if they are given when you are nearly fully dilated, or you are fully dilated (cervix open to 10 cm), they may not be as effective.

Anaesthetists (pain doctors) can be busy and will also need to see patients who are having a C-section first. Because of this and the fact it can take a long time to work, it's best to ask for an epidural early in labour if possible.

! It's best to ask for an epidural early in labour, as it may take a while for the specialist doctor (anaesthetist) to be free to see you and it takes 40 minutes to fully work.

An epidural blocks your pain from the top of your abdomen downwards. This means that if you have a long labour, it might let you sleep for a while.

? **How does the doctor do an epidural?**

They will:

- keep everything very clean (sterile) to make sure you don't get an infection
- ask you to either sit hugging your bump, or to lie on your side, to open up the lower back
- need you to be as still as you can, so tell them if you can feel a contraction building

- spray your back with a very cold cleaning spray – they will warn you before they do it
- give you some local pain relief through a needle into the skin – it can sting a bit, but will numb the skin so it hurts less to get the epidural
- then put the epidural in – you can feel pressure when they do this, and you might get a tingly sensation in one or both of your legs – tell them if this happens to you.

Once the epidural is working, you will still be able to feel pressure and touch, but not the pain.

You can watch an Autistic anaesthetist (pain doctor) talk about epidurals here:

What are the common side effects of an epidural?

- About one in every ten epidurals doesn't work perfectly – tell your health professional if you feel more pain on one side than the other or if you don't think your epidural is working.
- Many people feel sick – tell your health professional if this happens and they can give you some medication, or a bowl if you need to be sick.
- Your breathing might feel different to normal; some people feel breathless. Your doctors will be carefully monitoring your oxygen level, and they can give you extra oxygen through a mask or tube into your nose if you need it – tell your health professional if you feel breathless.
- You might feel itchy – tell your health professional if this is bothering you, as they might be able to change the medication.

- You might lose control of your bladder (pee yourself). Almost everyone will have a catheter put into their urethra (pee hole) to drain your bladder.
- You might not be able to tell when you're having a contraction. If this happens, a midwife will be able to help you know when to push.
- Your baby may have changes to their heartbeat, so it will be closely monitored.

If you are having an epidural or a top-up of your epidural medicine, continuous monitoring is recommended for a minimum of 30 minutes.

What Autistic people said... about epidurals

- Some people weren't sure whether to have one or not before labour, but had a lot of pain and found the epidural really helped.
- Some people knew they had a low pain tolerance, so decided they definitely wanted one before birth.
- Some people wanted an epidural, but they were too close to giving birth to have one.
- Some people chose not to have one because they wanted to be able to feel their contractions and follow their body's lead.
- Some people had an epidural with one or more of births, but not all of their births, as the pain level was different with each birth.
- People who had an epidural mostly said positive things, like how it made birth less painful, more relaxed and easier for them.

A 'spinal' (or spinal anaesthetic) is another type of pain relief that is similar to an epidural. It is a one-off injection into your back that gives pain relief for an hour or two. It tends to only be used for forceps or C-section births.

You can watch an Autistic parent talk about her experiences of having an epidural and a spinal block here:

If you've had an epidural, you'll need to rest in a lying or sitting position until the feeling comes back into your legs. This can take a few hours.

You can watch an Autistic doctor talk about what happens after birth if you've had an epidural here:

Things doctors can do to help deliver baby

Why might I need help from a doctor to deliver my baby?

Reasons about you

- You have a health condition, such as very high blood pressure, which may make pushing dangerous for you.
- You have been pushing for a long time and are very tired.
- Having an epidural has made it harder for you to push.

Reasons about your baby

- Your baby is premature (forceps can be safer than a vacuum cup).
- Your baby is in an awkward position.
- Your midwife or doctor think that baby needs to be delivered more quickly because there are concerns about their heart rate (they are 'in distress').

There are three main ways that doctors help to get babies out:

- making a cut between your vagina and anus to give more space (an episiotomy)
- using instruments to guide baby out through the vagina – these instruments are called forceps and vacuum cup (or ventouse)
- caesarean section, also called C-section.

We'll talk about each of these below.

Episiotomy

Episiotomies are when a doctor or midwife makes a cut to the area between the vagina and anus (the perineum).

This gives a bit of extra space to let baby be born. They are not routinely done in the UK, as it can take longer to heal from an episiotomy than if you tear during birth, but in some countries they are done for most births.

If you need a doctor to help deliver the baby using forceps or a vacuum cup, they will likely need to do an episiotomy first.

? Why are episiotomies (cuts to the genitals during birth) used?

They are usually used if baby is in distress or if it would be difficult or unsafe for you to give birth without one, including:

- if baby needs to be born quickly (when you are having a vaginal birth)
- to give more space to help with instrument deliveries, like using forceps
- if baby is being born bottom first or feet first (called a 'breech birth')
- if you have been pushing for a long time and are getting tired
- if you have a serious condition (like a known heart issue) that means it's safer for you not to be pushing for too long.

The health professionals should discuss this with you before doing anything.

Instrument-assisted delivery (forceps and ventouse)

A doctor will be called in if you need help to get baby out using instruments like forceps. If you have not had an epidural, you will usually be offered one.

The doctor will ask you to lie back, with your legs wide apart and your knees bent. Your legs and feet will be put in stirrups to raise them up (called the 'lithotomy position').

If baby is born using instruments, they may have small marks or bruises (including on their head and face). These are normal and will fade in a few days.

What are the different kinds of instruments used to help deliver baby and how are they used?

- **Forceps** are made of metal. They look a bit like a pair of large spoons or a pair of tongs. The bit that goes into your vagina is designed to fit around the baby's head.
- **Ventouse and Kiwi cup** are suction devices that work by making a vacuum seal on baby's head.

Using forceps or a vacuum cup, you will be asked to tell the doctor when you are having a contraction. If you've had an epidural, the midwife will watch the monitor or feel your tummy to tell you and the doctor when you're having a contraction.

They will ask you to push when they are ready. The doctor will then carefully and gently pull to help deliver your baby.

You can watch an Autistic doctor talk about what happens when forceps are used to try to deliver a baby here:

Caesarean section births

Sometimes it isn't possible to have a vaginal birth because of a complication, or sometimes you may choose to have a C-section. Getting baby out safely is the most important thing.

Around one in five births are by C-section.

Some parents choose to have a C-section before they give birth. This is also called an 'elective C-section'.

A C-section is major surgery to your tummy, and afterwards you have to be very careful how you move and might not be able to lift your baby. This can make it harder to breastfeed. You are generally not allowed to drive for 6–8 weeks after a C-section.

In the UK and many other countries, it is your decision if you want to have a C-section.

You can watch an Autistic midwife talk about choosing to have a C-section here:

What Autistic people said... about choosing to have a C-section

- Many parents who chose a C-section did it to reduce anxiety and increase control, especially if parents had already had a traumatic birth.
- Some parents had already had a C-section so were strongly recommended to have another one.
- Some parents whose babies were 'overdue' chose a C-section rather than being induced.
- Some babies were not in a good position for a natural birth (breech or back-to-back, where the back of baby's head and their back is against the parent's spine) or were large.

If you have had a C-section before this pregnancy, you might be told by your midwife or doctor that it is a good idea for you to have one to give birth again. But this isn't always the case, and some people give birth vaginally after a C-section.

> You can watch an Autistic parent talk about having an elective (planned) C-section here:

From start to finish, the whole thing takes around an hour. A lot of this is the preparation.

You will usually be allowed to have one birthing partner with you.

If you have an assistance dog with you at the hospital, they won't be allowed into the theatre, to keep everything sterile (very clean).

There will often be quite a lot of health professionals in the room. This can include:

- two or three doctors
- a midwife, midwifery support worker, and sometimes a student midwife
- an anaesthetist and an anaesthetics assistant
- one or two surgical nurses and sometimes theatre support workers.

If they are worried about you or baby being unwell, there may be more people than this.

You can ask for only essential staff to be in the operating room. You can also ask for them to only speak when needed.

> You can watch an Autistic doctor talk about what it's like going into an operating theatre, or operating room, here:

Most people who have a C-section are awake for it. This is known as having 'local anaesthetic'.

? What happens to get you ready to have a C-section?

- You will be in an operating room (also called an operating theatre).
- You will usually have an epidural for pain relief (see above).
- You will lie on a bed face-up, so you are looking at the ceiling. You may be able to see bright lights, medical equipment, and a cot for when your baby is born.
- A midwife, nurse or doctor will explain what will happen to you. They should give you time to ask questions.
- To top up your pain relief, you will usually have a cannula, a small tube into your bloodstream, put into the back of your hand if you don't already have one.
- You will have a catheter to drain urine from your bladder.
- To check that you are well, a health professional will connect some monitors to you. These are:
  - A blood pressure cuff on your arm. This will inflate with air at regular intervals, which can feel like it's squeezing your arm for a few seconds before the air goes out again.
  - An oxygen saturation probe on one of your fingers, which may feel a bit unusual, but shouldn't hurt. It also measures your pulse.
  - Some small sticky pads on your chest (this can include under your breast), arms and legs, connected to leads to be able to monitor your heart.
- A screen or fabric sheet will be put up between your head and your tummy, so you won't see the operation.
- The anaesthetist (pain relief doctor) will be near your head, and they will monitor you closely during the surgery. You can speak to them if you have any worries about anything.

- Sometimes the bed will be tilted slightly, to reduce the pressure from your baby bump, which can make you feel sick.

Once everything has been set up, the operation will start. This is usually quite quick – up to 20 minutes.

You can watch an Autistic doctor talk about everything to do with having a C-section here:

Occasionally, they may need to give you a general anaesthetic to do a C-section. This would usually be in the rare case of a spinal anesthetic or epidural not working well enough, or not being suitable for you. Rarely it would be because the doctors are very worried about you or your baby and there isn't time to do an epidural. You can ask your midwife what would happen in the hospital you are giving birth in.

You can watch an Autistic doctor talk about having a general anaesthetic for a C-section here:

What happens to get the baby out during a C-section?

- A cut is made in your tummy and womb. This is usually horizontal (going across the body) below your bikini line.
- Getting the baby out of your tummy can feel very strange, with sensations including pushing, pulling, tugging and stretching. Some people don't feel anything.
- It shouldn't be painful – let the doctor or nurses know if you are in pain; they can give you more pain relief.

You can see a drawing of what happens during a C-section here:

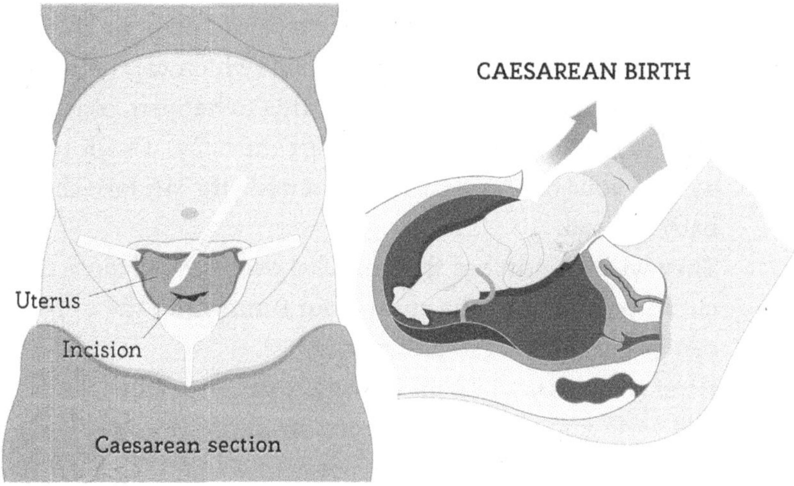

A drawing of a caesarean birth

When the baby is born, you will stay in the operating room for a bit longer.

What happens straight after the baby is born during a C-section?

- When the baby is born, some will cry straight away, but it's also normal for the baby not to cry straight away.
- The surgeons will usually hold the baby up for you to see.
- There are then two options:
  - If the baby is a bit shocked by being born, it will go straight to the midwives who can give some extra help. This is quite common with caesarean section births and not something you need to worry about.
  - If the baby is well, the surgeon will usually rest the baby between your legs for a few minutes with the umbilical cord still attached to get all of the blood from the cord before giving baby to the midwives.
- You're usually given an injection of oxytocin, to reduce blood loss.

- The doctors will remove your placenta from the womb.
- Once the baby has been dried and the midwives and doctors are happy, the baby will be placed on your chest. This can include having skin-to-skin (which can help with breastfeeding). If you don't want this to happen, or if you start to feel uncomfortable holding the baby, it's OK to say so, and your birthing partner or a midwife can take the baby instead.
- They will use stitches that dissolve over time to close the cut in your womb. The cut in your tummy (on the outside) can be closed with staples or stitches.
- After this, they will help you safely get onto a bed, and will wash you to clean you from the surgery.

What Autistic people said... about having a C-section

- People generally didn't feel surprised about anything that happened.
- The tugging feeling of getting baby out was weird.
- Some people found being awake but not able to move whilst feeling the tugging traumatic.
- Some people liked everything about it.
- Some people found the sensory experience of being in the operating room was better than expected.
- Some people had weird skin sensations or itchiness around their scar afterwards.
- Some people felt funny from the anaesthetic.
- People who needed an emergency C-section sometimes said everything happened in a rush without much explanation, which was worrying, but they felt confident in the health professionals around them.

Birth plan – part 2

We started to look at what goes on a birth plan in the previous chapter (Chapter 8). The section below covers the things we've talked about in this chapter. You can put it together with your decisions from Chapter 8. There will be more decisions to make in Chapter 10. A downloadable version of the full birth plan for you to fill out yourself can be found at www.jkp.com/catalogue/book/9781839978609, as indicated by a symbol.

Tool: Birth plan part 2 – giving birth and pain relief

Decision to be made	Choices
Checking my labour progress	
Touching my tummy (to check your contractions)	I do not want my tummy to be touched to check my contractions
	I need to be asked and have time to decide each time you want to touch my tummy to check my contractions
	I am happy for you to touch my tummy to check my contractions
Vaginal exams (to check your cervix)	Please tell me if you think it is an emergency and you really need to do a vaginal exam. You still need to wait for me to consent.
	I do not want vaginal exams
	I want to wait and see what happens when giving birth
	I can do my own vaginal exam
	I agree to vaginal exams, but want to be asked for consent every time
	I only want female midwives and doctors to do vaginal exams
	Only women staff to do vaginal examinations unless it's urgently needed
	I have had bad experiences in the past and I will need extra time and patience
	If it hurts, I need you to stop immediately
	No repeat vaginal examinations (eg: by the midwife and then the doctor)

cont.

Decision to be made	Choices
Communicating about birth progressing and pain	
Moving into established labour or time to push	I am likely to be quiet and calm even when I'm in a lot of pain
	I might become overwhelmed and stop being able to speak
	Please can you check my cervix for progress if you don't believe me when I say I think my birth is progressing
	If I say I am in pain, please believe me and provide more pain relief if it is safe
Monitoring baby	
Continuous monitoring (usually using wires)	I prefer not to have continuous monitoring if possible
	I would prefer to have telemetry (no wires) if available
	Continuous monitoring using bands around my belly is OK for me
	Continuous monitoring including a small clip on baby's head is OK for me
Taking a tiny blood sample from baby's scalp during birth (foetal blood sampling)	I don't want foetal blood sampling
	I'm happy to have foetal blood sampling if it is needed
When it's time to push	
Helping me know when it's time	I'm worried that I won't know when to push
	Can you check where baby's head is to let me know if it's time?
When I'm pushing	I don't want you to talk to me unless necessary
	I would like you to encourage me
	Please say this to encourage me (write your answer)
	Please don't say this (write your answer)
If I look like I'm running out of energy	I want you to encourage me if you think birth will happen soon
	I want you to offer me assistance from a doctor to get baby out

My pain relief plan	
I want to use Check if the midwife or hospital has these or if you can bring your own.	Natural methods, like hypnobirthing or aromatherapy
	A water birth
	A birthing ball
	An active birth room
	My birth partner massaging me
	A warm cloth on the perinium
	TENS machine
	Paracetamol
	Gas and air
	Injected medication
	Epidural
	I would like anti-sickness medication with injected medicine or an epidural
I do not want any medication	Please do not offer me any pain relief
Extra help to get baby out	
Episiotomy (being cut)	I do not want to be cut – I will tear naturally if needed
	I agree to be cut if it's needed – please make sure I consent at the time
	I need pain relief in the area (local anaesthetic injection) before you make the cut
If baby needs to be born urgently	It is important that you tell me what you are going to do before you do it and get my consent
	I am happy for you to try using things like forceps or suction cup (ventouse) through my vagina
	I would like you to show me the forceps or suction cup (ventouse) before you use it, unless it is an emergency
	I would prefer a C-section
	If I need a cannula (tube in my hand) for medication, please put it in my (choose: left or right) hand

An Autistic midwife's top tips... on giving birth and pain relief

By Diane Fox, RM, PGCPSE PGDPSE

- Complete your birth plan outlining your pain relief preferences and preferences for assisted delivery.
- Add your preferences in emergencies for sensory and communication needs to your birth plan.
- Advise your health professionals if you want your partner to advocate for you as you may be unable to fully process and communicate sometimes.
- Be vocal about if you are in pain. Just in case this is difficult, consider having signals with your partner, such as a hand signal, to indicate if you need more pain relief, so you don't have to use words or explain. Or you might want to have sentences pre-written and point to them. Then your partner can advocate for you or you can show them directly to the midwife.
- If having a C-section, if you need anything in the theatre ask the anaesthetist (who will be stood or sat near your head) to communicate to other staff your needs on your behalf.
- In emergencies things can move fast but it will be over quickly and you will soon be united with your baby.
- Ask for a full debrief after the emergency if you can process it at the time. If not, you can ask for this at a later date.
- Once back home, tell your midwife/health visitor or GP if you feel negatively affected by the events around birth or found it traumatic, to access support and treatment as soon as possible. Autistic people can have a higher incidence of postnatal depression and post-traumatic stress disorder (PTSD).

Conclusion

You've made it to the end of Chapter 9! We've covered lots of things to do with baby being born. This includes the different stages of labour, monitoring you and baby during birth, pain and pain relief, and doctors helping baby be born by C-section or using forceps. I hope this helps to give you an idea of what might happen, but if you're worried about anything, please speak to your midwife or health professional. Next, we'll be thinking about what happens immediately after baby is born – there are some more decisions to be made and it might be helpful for you to think about these in advance, although it's OK for you to go to whatever section you like.

CHAPTER 10

Immediately After Baby Is Born

CONTENTS

Introduction

This is the third and final chapter focused on what happens when you give birth.

We start this chapter thinking about 'the golden hour', which is a name given to the first hour after baby has been born.

After this, we talk about the post-birth examination you'll be offered to check if you have any tears to your genitals. We'll also think about the treatment options, including stitches.

We'll then think about what happens on the postnatal ward, and going home.

Finally, there is some information about making a complaint if things went wrong whilst you were giving birth.

The golden hour: the first 60 minutes after birth

A lot happens in the first hour after birth, and it can feel really busy and overwhelming.

There are lots of things that you might want to make decisions about before you give birth, including adding them to your birth plan if you make one. This can make it feel less stressful when you are asked questions.

What Autistic people said... about what happened straight after birth

- They could feel overstimulated and overwhelmed if they were in hospital, as they became more aware of the busyness around them.
- They could feel relaxed and comfortable at home (although if there were complications during birth, they had to transfer to hospital).
- If they'd had an epidural it could be a while before their legs were ready for them to stand, which could feel weird and tingly.
- Some people who had a catheter (to have an epidural or

C-section) had this left in for a long time because the nurses were busy, which made it difficult to get around.
- Some people needed treatment like stitches or medicine for heavy bleeding (talked about more below).

Delayed cord clamping and cutting the cord

Leaving the umbilical cord, which connects the baby and the placenta, in place for a short time after birth is recommended. It stays attached to baby without being 'clamped' or cut until it stops pulsing. This is known as **delayed cord clamping** or **deferred cord clamping**.

This lets all of the blood in the placenta go into the baby. The extra blood helps to increase baby's iron, helping with growth, and gives them extra stem cells, which helps their immune system.

It usually takes a few minutes.

If you do delayed cord clamping, the baby will still be attached to the placenta, which is still in your uterus, with the cord being in your vagina if you had a vaginal delivery. This means you and baby need to stay close to each other, and it may be difficult for someone else to hold them.

If you had a C-section, the surgeons will carefully put baby between your legs if you do delayed cord clamping, unless it is an emergency, when they would be unable to do it.

Giving baby vitamin K

As soon as your baby is born, you will be asked if you want them to have a vitamin K injection. Another option is to have oral drops. It's best to decide this in advance, so you don't have to rush your decision.

? What is vitamin K, and why might my baby need it?

- Vitamin K is part of the blood clotting process.
- Babies only have a tiny amount of vitamin K when they are born.
- This means they have an increased risk of having a very rare condition where, as well as bleeding from any cuts or grazes, they could bleed into their intestines or

brain, which can be very serious, including death. This is called 'haemorrhagic disease of the newborn', 'vitamin K deficiency bleeding' or VKDB.

- Having an injection of vitamin K reduces the risk of this type of bleeding.
- Another option is for baby to have oral drops twice in their first week and once at one month of age. The downside of oral drops is if baby is sick, they might not absorb the vitamin K.

Delivering the placenta (the third stage of labour)

If you have a C-section, the doctors will have removed your placenta in the operating room.

After you have given birth vaginally, it can take up to an hour for the placenta to come away from the wall of your uterus naturally (by itself). This is also called a 'physiological third stage'.

When this happens you will usually feel some pressure in your bottom. You will then push it out, and it should only take a few minutes for you to 'deliver' the placenta. It usually isn't painful (it's much smaller than your baby).

You may be offered an injection of synthetic oxytocin, including the drugs ergometrine or Syntocinon. These can speed up how quickly the placenta detaches. If you agree to this, the midwife will inject you in your thigh as soon as you give birth.

This will make your womb contract, and the placenta will come away from your womb in around five to ten minutes. When this happens, the midwife will press on your tummy from above and gently pull the cord to pull the placenta out through your vagina. This is called 'active management'.

There are pros and cons to having an oxytocin injection. The UK NHS says it reduces the risk of heavy bleeding (post-partum haemorrhage) but increases the chances of you feeling sick and vomiting. You can have an anti-sickness injection if needed. It can also make afterpains feel more intense.

We talk more about heavy bleeding and afterpains later in the chapter.

Skin-to-skin contact

Skin-to-skin means putting your naked baby against your bare chest (it's OK to have a blanket or clean towel over the top of both of you). If you do this, you will naturally get an increase in a hormone called oxytocin.

If baby is left in skin-to-skin without being interrupted (by partners or health professionals), they will have their first breastfeed. This can take some time, with baby stopping and resting when needed.

What are the benefits of skin-to-skin?

- Calms you and baby; the pressure of baby on your chest may also feel nice from a sensory point of view.
- Helps to regulate baby's heartbeat.
- Controls baby's temperature.
- Lowers the risk of baby getting an infection, as they pick up healthy bacteria from your skin.
- Releases your hormones to support breastfeeding and nurturing.
- Boosts baby's digestion and interest in feeding.
- There are extra benefits for babies who are premature or in the neonatal unit, including reducing stress and improving the amount of oxygen in their blood.

You can watch an Autistic antenatal educator talk about skin-to-skin here:

What Autistic people said... about skin-to-skin after birth

- Many parents really enjoyed skin-to-skin.
- Sometimes health professionals didn't help to do skin-to-skin, which meant the parent might need to push for this to happen.

- Some parents felt really sensitive to touch in their pregnancy and didn't want to do skin-to-skin.
- Some **really, really** didn't want to do it.
- Whatever their decision, making sure their birthing partner knew this ahead of time made them less worried about their wishes being followed.

Before you give birth, decide if you want baby to have a vitamin K injection, if you want an injection to help deliver the placenta, and if you want to do 'skin-to-skin' with baby. Tell your birthing partner or midwife, so they can help you get the care you want.

The first feed

We'll talk more about feeding baby in Chapter 11, but it's relevant to think about baby's first feed here. If you are breastfeeding and able to do skin-to-skin without interruption, baby may be able to latch onto the breast themselves and feed.

If there are interruptions, it may be harder for baby, and many new parents find breastfeeding difficult. If you want to breastfeed and you aren't sure how things are going, it's OK to ask for help.

Script: Things to say when you're doing or want to do skin-to-skin

- 'Does this look OK for skin-to-skin?'
- 'I want to do skin-to-skin, but we've had some interruptions and I don't know if baby is finding their way to feed. Does it look OK to you?'
- (If a health professional goes to disturb baby) 'I'm doing skin-to-skin and it hasn't been an hour yet. Would it be OK to give us some more time?'
- (If your partner goes to pick up baby) 'Please don't. Do you remember, skin-to-skin is really important for baby's health? Can you wait until they've had their first feed and then you can hold them?'

Tears during birth and the post-birth examination

During birth many people will experience a graze or tear to the skin of the inner labia (labia minora). Some will have a tear to the outer labia (labia majora) or may tear muscles inside their vagina or tear between the vagina and anus.

After birth you will be offered a vaginal examination by your midwife or obstetrician, to see if you have any tears. They will then let you know if you need any stitches (sutures). Stitches are needed to prevent infection if the tear is bleeding or if it includes the anus. If there is a tear between the vagina and anus, stitches are very important as otherwise you could pass poo without meaning to (have faecal incontinence).

After birth you will be asked to have an examination of your genitals to see if you have any injuries from birth ('tears'). You may be offered stitches if the tear is bleeding or includes your anus.

You can watch an Autistic midwife talk about the after birth examination, tears and stitches here:

How can I get ready for the post-birth examination?

- If you are in pain, you can request painkillers before they examine you, and you can request this part way through the examination too.
- You can use gas and air.
- You can always ask them to stop at any point during the examination.
- You can ask them to talk to you as they go along, such as telling you:
  - what they are about to do
  - what they have found.

- Or, you can ask them not to talk to you until the end if you prefer.
- Stimming and distraction may help you cope during the examination, but it might be helpful to tell the person doing the exam what you'll do first.
- If you lose speech during painful procedures, you may want to have somebody present with you, or some other ways to communicate, such as tapping them and holding a hand up to request for the examination to stop.

It might also make you feel more comfortable to know what to expect. The midwife should tell you what's going to happen, but some parents have said that they were surprised by some of the examinations.

What is included in the post birth examination?

The examination may include the midwife:

- asking you to open your legs

Part 1: Vulva

- looking at your vulva with a light
- washing your vulva with warm water and looking to see if there are any tears or grazes on the outside.

Part 2: Vagina

- gently parting your vulva to look inside the vagina
- wiping away any bleeding with gauze.

Part 3: Rectum (anus and 'back passage') and vagina together

- inserting one finger into your anus and one finger into your vagina at the same time
- checking for any tears between the vagina and rectum.

This is important to make sure no poo (faeces) can get into the vagina from the rectum.

If you have any tears, the midwife will discuss a treatment plan with you.

Your midwife might recommend treatment to you after the exam. As always, you don't have to have this treatment, but if you have a second-, third- or fourth-degree tear it can be really important for your long-term health.

What do the different degrees of tears mean and how are they treated?

First-degree tear: These are small grazes or tears that only impact the **skin**. They can be very sore.

- They only need stitches if they're bleeding.
- They usually heal quickly and without medical treatment.
- Wash or shower at least once a day.
- Only use water to keep the area clean.
- Change your sanitary pads regularly.
- You can pour water over yourself as you pee if it stings.

Second-degree tear: These impact the **skin and muscles** of the vagina and often need stitches. Midwives will usually repair these in the room you are in.

- They may need you to open your legs wide or put them into stirrups.
- They will give you a 'local anaesthetic': an injection of painkiller into the area to make it go numb.
- Then they will use a small needle and surgical thread to bring the sides of the tear together.
- If you feel any pain, ask for more pain relief.
- The stitches will dissolve within a few weeks.

- You will have another examination in a few weeks to make sure the tear has healed fully.

Third-degree tear: The tear affects the **vagina and anus**. These often need to be repaired in an operating theatre by a doctor.

Fourth-degree tear: These are rare. They are similar to a third-degree tear but go further into the **lining of your anus or bowel**. These will need to be repaired in an operating theatre by a doctor.

Some people feel pain or discomfort after their stitches. As well as painkillers, you may find that a cool (not frozen) sanitary pad or a warm bath can give some relief.

? **What are the signs something is wrong with my stitches?**

If you have stitches, you can get an infection. Symptoms of this include:

- a lot of pain in the area where the stitches are
- a discharge that smells different to normal, including smelling really bad ('foul smelling')
- a raised temperature
- feeling unwell
- increased bleeding.

If you have any of these, you should contact your midwife or GP, as you may need treatment (such as antibiotics). If you are unable to get an appointment with your midwife or GP and have any worries, contact your local maternity unit.

! If you have any worries about your stitches, like pain, discharge or bleeding, or you have a temperature, contact your midwife, GP or local maternity unit.

What Autistic people said... about having stitches

- Most didn't say anything positive or negative about the exam or getting stitches.
- Some people had a bad experience, with pain during the exam or when getting stitches, and midwives who were unsympathetic to their pain or wouldn't give enough pain relief.
- Some people didn't know how to take care of their stitches and found it hard to get information from midwives.

You can watch an Autistic parent talk about their experience of having stitches here:

Heavy vaginal bleeding after birth ('postpartum haemorrhage')

After you've given birth, there is a risk of heavy bleeding from the vagina for the first 12 weeks. This happens to between 1 in 20 or 1 in 33 (3%–5%) of people.

In the 24 hours after you've given birth, losing over a pint (or 500 ml) of blood is classed as 'heavy'. If you are bleeding a lot you might also feel dizzy, sick or light-headed.

Let your health professionals know if you have heavy bleeding or any of these symptoms. If you are unsure if your blood loss is 'heavy', ask them – don't wait to see if it gets worse.

! If you are bleeding after birth and don't know if it's 'too much' or 'heavy bleeding' ask your midwife.

If you have heavy bleeding, it is a medical emergency and you need to let a health professional know urgently.

If they are worried about your blood loss, they will get to work straight away to stop the bleeding.

If you have heavy bleeding after birth this is a medical emergency – get medical help urgently.

How is heavy bleeding on the day after birth treated?

If you are in the first 24 hours after birth, your midwife or doctor will:

- Monitor your blood pressure, breathing, oxygen level and other vital signs (see Chapter 6, pages 120–121, for details).
- Keep you on the labour ward until the bleeding slows down.
- If you have a home birth or give birth in a birthing centre, you will be transferred to hospital.
- If they decide you need treatment, they should tell you exactly what they're going to do. If you are looking very unwell, they might tell you quickly and start treating you.

They might:

- Massage your womb, through your tummy or vagina.
- Give you medicine to reduce the bleeding. This can be as an IV drip or an injection into your thigh.
- Put a small tube ('catheter') into your bladder to empty it.
- Give you fluids through an IV drip.

If the bleeding doesn't stop, you might also need:

- a blood transfusion
- surgery under general anaesthetic to find out why you are bleeding heavily and stop the bleeding.

If you've had heavy bleeding after birth, it can be frightening, as the staff are suddenly very busy around you.

When you are stable – the bleeding has slowed down – you should be able to talk to a doctor or senior midwife about what has happened ('have a debrief'). They should go through each step and explain it to you.

If you have heavy bleeding more than 24 hours after birth but within the first three months, this can be a sign of an infection in your womb. You might also notice a bad smell in your vaginal blood or feel unwell. Try to remember these signs of infection, and seek medical help if you have any of them.

! If your vaginal blood smells bad, you feel unwell or you have heavy bleeding in the first three months after birth, speak to your midwife or doctor as you might have an infection.

If you have had heavy bleeding in the past, you are more likely to have it if you give birth again. Because of this, the doctors will likely suggest you give birth in hospital. They will also take extra steps to monitor and treat you.

What happens after the first hour?

If you gave birth on a ward or midwifery-led unit, you'll usually be able to stay there for a few hours. This gives you time to have uninterrupted 'skin-to-skin' time with baby, something to eat and drink, and time for a shower.

If you have an agreed 'reasonable adjustment' to have a room by yourself on the postnatal ward, they may let you stay on the delivery ward until there is a room available. You should always ask about this before you give birth.

After this, you'll usually be taken to the postnatal ward. Sometimes if you have an uncomplicated vaginal birth, you can go home afterwards instead of going to the postnatal ward. This would usually be a minimum of six hours after you give birth (see the section 'When will I be able to go home after birth?' below).

If you gave birth in the operating theatre, such as to have a C-section, you will usually go straight to the recovery area or postnatal ward. They can help you to have skin-to-skin contact if you like.

The postnatal ward

Most postnatal wards in the UK have 'bays' with more than one bed per room. Often there are four to six parents and their babies in each of the bays. There will be a bathroom or several bathrooms to share.

There is no standard rule about whether you should or shouldn't take your baby (in their crib) to the toilet with you, and what to do when you want to take a shower.

If you have a birthing partner with you on the ward who can watch the baby, it's fine to leave them with baby. If you are alone, it is best to ask the midwives what they would prefer you to do, as they may not want babies to be left unattended. You can ask once and then do what they said each time, unless you are told something different.

There are also sometimes a smaller number of single rooms. These are used for mums who have complications or additional needs. If they have them in your hospital, you can ask if you would be able to have one. It's best to talk to your midwife about this before you give birth. Some hospitals in the UK let you pay to use a side room if there is one not being used.

You may find that being on the postnatal ward seems quite different to what you expected.

You can watch an Autistic parent talk about how the postnatal ward was different to what they expected from TV shows here:

How can I get help on the postnatal ward?

Often you will be given a 'call bell' that looks a bit like a TV remote control connected to the wall with a wire. The staff should show you how to use it, but generally you can press it to ask a midwife to come and help you. Sometimes if the midwives are busy, it may take a long time for someone to answer when you 'buzz'.

If there is a midwife or other health professional in the room who's just finished helping somebody else, you could ask them, 'Excuse me, could you help me?'

Each ward will have a 'midwives' station' with computers which is where the midwives tend to be when they are doing paperwork and between helping patients. If something is urgent, like you have started to bleed a lot or you are worried about baby, you could go to the midwives' station (if you are safe to walk) or see if somebody (a cleaner or other parent) could get a midwife for you.

All parents can find being on the postnatal ward busy and loud, and they might find it hard to know how to ask for help. But, it can be useful to be around so many health professionals too. Staff can also help you with feeding, whether you want to breast or formula feed. They can also help you if you are worried about anything to do with your baby.

! When you're in hospital, if you are worried about baby or yourself, ask a midwife for help. If you are very worried, such as if you are heavily bleeding or baby seems unwell, see if another parent can get a midwife for you.

? **What will the midwives and doctors do on the postnatal ward?**

Whilst you're in hospital, midwives will check your 'observations' (also called 'vital observations'), like your temperature, blood pressure, pulse and oxygen level in your blood (see Chapter 6, pages 120–121), at regular intervals. This should only take a few minutes each time. It might be a midwifery support worker who does this, rather than a qualified midwife.

Midwives

Each day that you are on the postnatal ward, you should be seen by a midwife. They will ask you things like:

- how much you're bleeding from your vagina (they may ask to see your sanitary pad)
- if you have any pain in your tummy, vagina or stitches
- if there's any pain or tenderness in your breasts and nipples
- about your sleep and mood
- if you feel like you're bonding with baby
- how much you've been going to the toilet (for a wee and a poo)
- if you have any pain or swelling in your legs
- anything else you're concerned about, physically and emotionally.

They will also want to:

- feel your tummy, to check your womb; if this hurts, let them know
- check your C-section incision if you had one.

They will also check baby, including:

- asking you how baby is feeding
- asking you how many wet and dirty nappies baby has had, and the colour of their poo
- taking off baby's clothes and checking they are physically well
- asking if you have any concerns about anything.

If anything feels difficult or you're worried about anything, let them know.

Doctors

The doctors usually visit the ward in the morning. There are two types of doctors: obstetricians oversee the care of those who gave birth, and paediatricians oversee the care of babies.

They will ask the midwives about which parents and babies need to be seen by them. If the midwives are happy that you and baby are well, you might not have a doctor come to see you.

If the midwives have any worries at any time (day or night), they can call a doctor to check on you or your baby.

You can watch an Autistic midwife talk about what happens on the postnatal ward here:

If you're finding it really hard to be in hospital because of the sensory environment, you could ask if it would be safe for you to go home.

When will I be able to go home after birth?

There's no set time for when you will be able to go home.

Before you can go home, the midwives and doctors will want to make sure:

- your bleeding is normal (not heavy)
- you've had a wee
- baby is feeding well
- baby has been checked head-to-toe by the children's doctors (paediatricians)
- baby has had a wee and poo
- you and baby seem well.

If you had a straightforward vaginal birth, this could be within six to ten hours after you give birth. Occasionally you might be able to go home and bring baby back so you can be checked by the children's doctors (paediatricians) the next day.

If you had a C-section it can be a few days.

You can watch an Autistic parent share their experience of staying on the postnatal ward here:

Early treatment after having a stressful birth

If you found your birth stressful or traumatic, some research suggests that playing a video game like Tetris on your phone soon after (up to 6 hours) can reduce the trauma later on.

You can also ask your midwife to have a discussion about your birth.

Changes to your body after birth

In this chapter, we'll just think about things that happen in the tummy and genital area. In the next chapter we think about changes to your breasts.

'Afterpains' – your womb shrinking back to its usual size

After you give birth, your womb will shrink back to its usual size. It can take six weeks for this to happen.

Some people find that they get 'afterpains' with this. They can be like period pains or like less strong contractions. They usually stop after three days.

You can watch an Autistic lactation consultant talk about afterpains here:

What treatment is available for afterpains?

- Painkillers like paracetamol or ibuprofen.
- Drink lots of water.

- Pee more often, as a full bladder can make it worse.
- Heat pads or hot water bottles on your tummy or back.

If these don't work for you, phone your midwife and tell them, as you might have an infection.

You can watch an Autistic parent talk about their experience of very painful afterpains here:

Going to the toilet

If you find peeing hurts your skin, drinking lots can dilute your urine to make it sting less. You can also pour water on yourself as you pee to help with stinging. If you're finding it hard to pee, it's very sore or you notice a bad smell, tell your midwife.

The first poo after birth can feel painful (and worrying!). Try not to strain.

If you have stitches, you might worry about having a poo but it's **very unlikely** they will open from you having a poo. You can gently hold a clean sanitary pad or some clean toilet paper against the area between your vagina and bum (your perineum) to give you more control over how quickly the poo comes out. If you're leaking poo, or pooing when you don't mean to, tell your midwife or doctor.

It's very unlikely your stitches will open from having a poo, but try to poo slowly if you're worried. Holding gentle pressure against the area between your vagina and bum hole can give you more control over the speed.

How soon after birth can I use tampons or a menstrual cup?

You shouldn't use tampons or any other menstrual product that goes inside your vagina until after your six-week postnatal check-up.

This is because using 'internal' menstrual products gives a bigger risk of getting an infection.

This means the only safe menstrual product is a pad that you place in your underwear.

What if things went wrong with your care?

In Chapter 9 we talked about complaining or asking for better care when you were in hospital.

There will be a formal way of making a complaint about medical treatment in your country. You should be able to find information about this online by searching for the name of your country and 'maternity care complaint'.

You can watch an Autistic parent talk about the process of making a formal complaint about maternity care in the UK here:

Sometimes submitting a complaint will take a lot of energy, so don't feel bad if you decide not to.

Birth plan - part 3

We started to look at what goes on a birth plan in Chapter 8, and looked at more options in Chapter 9. The section below covers the things we've talked about in this chapter. You can put it together with your decisions from Chapters 8 and 9. A downloadable version of the full birth plan for you to fill out yourself can be found at www.jkp.com/catalogue/book/9781839978609, as indicated by a ✱ symbol.

Tool: Birth plan part 3 – what happens after birth

Decisions for the hour after birth	
Cord clamping	I want delayed cord cutting (including if I have a caesarean)
	I want me or my birthing partner to cut the cord
	I want a health professional to cut the cord
Vitamin K injection for baby	I want baby to have the vitamin K injection
	I want baby to have vitamin K drops (by mouth)
	I don't want baby to have vitamin K
Delivering the placenta	I want to naturally deliver the placenta, unless there is a medical emergency
	I want to be given an oxytocin injection in my thigh to speed up delivering the placenta
If I bleed heavily after birth	I understand that I may need extra medicines. If I am very unwell or unconscious, the midwives and doctors will make decisions for me.
	If there is time, I would like you to explain your decisions to me and ask for my agreement ('consent')
	I would like to talk to a midwife or doctor after treatment (have a 'debrief') to understand what happened
Skin-to-skin and feeding baby after birth	I want skin-to-skin contact with baby
	Only talk to me if necessary whilst I'm having skin-to-skin
	I want to breastfeed
	I want to formula feed
After-birth genital examination, tears and stitches	
Doing the exam	I'm worried about the post-birth examination and if I need to have stitches – please tell me what you're going to do before you do it
	If I am in pain, I will need you to stop and get more pain relief before you can continue
	I would like you to tell me what you've found as you are doing the examination
	I would like you to wait until the end of the examination to tell me what you've found

cont.

Feeding	
Getting help with feeding baby	I'm not sure how to get baby latched on to breastfeed – please can I have some help
	Please use a hands-off (not touching me) way of showing me things
	Please don't touch me without asking first
	I'm not sure how to make a bottle of formula – can you please help me?
	I'm not sure how to feed baby using a bottle – can you please help?
	I don't know how to 'wind' or 'burp' my baby – can you please show me?
After labour ward	
Location	I would like to go home as soon as possible after birth if it's safe
	I will go to the postnatal ward
	I would like a side room on the postnatal ward – **tell your midwife this in a routine pregnancy appointment**

An Autistic midwife's top tips... on the time straight after you give birth

By Diane Fox, RM, PGCPSE PGDPSE

- Use the BRAIN tool (see Chapter 8, page 177) to consider the pros and cons of baby having a vitamin K injection, active management of the third stage of labour and delivering the placenta.
- Ensure a plan is in place for a single room if you need one on the postnatal ward.
- Ensure you have enough pain relief for internal examinations and perinatal repair if needed.
- Ask about what options are available to go home quickly if you need to because of sensory overwhelm or overload.
- Ask for a key person to support you on every shift on the postnatal ward so you can go directly to them for help and support as needed.

Conclusion

You've made it to the end of Chapter 10! We've covered everything to do with what happens straight after you've given birth. A lot happens in the first hour, including some decisions for you to make in advance, like if you want to delay cord clamping, if you want your baby to have vitamin K, if you want medication to help deliver the placenta, and if you want to have skin-to-skin contact with baby. There are no right or wrong answers for these. We also thought about the check of your genitals the midwife does after birth, treatment if you have any tears, and changes to your genitals after birth. Remember, as always, if you're worried about anything, please speak to your midwife or health professional. Next, we'll be thinking about some of the key bits of looking after a new baby: sleep, crying and feeding. But it's OK for you to go to whatever section you like.

SECTION III

THE FOURTH TRIMESTER (WHEN BABY HAS ARRIVED)

CHAPTER 11

Sleep, Crying and Feeding Your Baby

CONTENTS

Introduction

When it comes to looking after your baby, there is rarely a single right answer. Instead, decisions will come down to what suits you and your family.

We start off by talking about sleep, including normal baby sleeping patterns, sudden infant death syndrome (SIDS) and co-sleeping.

We then think about the reasons baby cries, how to soothe them, and colic.

Next, we talk about the safe ways to feed your baby. From birth until they are six months old, babies only need to be fed breast- or formula milk, and shouldn't have any other drinks or food.

Although feeding a baby sounds simple, many parents find it can be difficult, and some parents can be very worried about it. I will share the basics of the most important things you need to know.

We then think about normal baby feeding patterns and common worries about feeding babies.

Sleep

Normal baby sleep

It's very normal for newborn babies to sleep a lot. Sometimes this is in short stretches and other times they are longer, up to around four hours at most. Often it may seem that they sleep randomly, with no fixed pattern. This is all normal (even if it's difficult for parents).

Below three months of age, babies won't sleep through the night. This is because a new baby's tummy is small, so they **need** to be fed often. They also sleep lightly, so can be woken up easily.

Sometimes newborn babies tend to sleep more in the day and less at night. This is because breastmilk-making hormones are highest at night, so babies know to feed more then. Also, they don't yet know the difference between day and night.

In total, newborn babies tend to sleep for between 8 and 20 hours per day. There's a big variation in time there, but it's entirely down to your baby how much they sleep, and either is completely normal.

What Autistic people said... about newborn baby sleep

- It was common to feel extremely tired, and this could continue for several months with babies waking every few hours overnight.
- If they had a partner who worked, it could feel even worse when their partner went back to work.
- Sometimes parents were so tired they fell asleep when holding their baby, which they knew was unsafe and worried them.
- Taking shifts with their partner (or a trusted friend, family member or doula) helped them to get some good-quality sleep.
- Some partners would agree to take baby for a shift but refuse to wake up to care for the baby, which was frustrating and upsetting.
- Some parents said that focusing on doing the bare minimum around the house and saying no to unhelpful visitors so they could sleep helped.
- Several people noted that this phase didn't last forever, and it made them feel better to think that way.

Safer sleep and sudden infant death syndrome (SIDS)

It's safest for new babies to sleep in their own cot or Moses basket in the same room as you. This is for both naps and overnight.

They should be put to sleep on their back. This is because it reduces the risk of sudden infant death syndrome (SIDS), where otherwise healthy babies suddenly die.

What is sudden infant death syndrome (SIDS)?

Sudden infant death syndrome, or SIDS, is when a baby who is healthy suddenly dies without a clear reason.

SIDS often happens when babies are sleeping.

There are some risk factors for when SIDS is more likely. We will talk about those and how you can reduce the risk of SIDS below.

Safer co-sleeping and SIDS

Co-sleeping is sharing a bed with your baby or child. Many parents find co-sleeping helps the family to get more sleep. It can also help with breastfeeding when baby is feeding a lot, as you can lie down whilst baby feeds.

If you don't plan to co-sleep, you might still fall asleep whilst feeding or soothing baby. For that reason, the Lullaby Trust recommend that all parents make their beds as safe as possible for baby.

? How can I make my bed safer to co-sleep?

This advice is given because SIDS is more likely if you share a bed with your baby.

- Keep all bedding and pillows away from where they could accidentally cover the baby when you are asleep.
- If you get cold overnight, sleep wearing warm clothes instead of relying on bedding to keep you warm.
- Don't have other children or pets in the bed, as they could accidentally harm the baby.
- Make sure your baby:
  - is lying on their back
  - can't get trapped between the mattress and the wall (or anything else)
  - can't fall out of the bed.

? How can I reduce the risk of sudden infant death syndrome (SIDS)?

Because SIDS often happens when babies are sleeping, the advice focuses on sleep.

You can **reduce** the risk of SIDS by baby sleeping:

- On their back – not their stomach or side.
- On a firm, flat and waterproof mattress – not a soft surface like a fluffy blanket, soft mattress or waterbed.
- In their own cot or bassinet in the same room as their

parents – not sharing a bed with parents, and especially not with other children or pets.

- Keep the cot as bare as possible – no pillows, toys or fluffy blankets.
- With their feet at the end of the cot, to stop them wriggling down under the covers.
- In a room that's around 16–20 °C – if babies get too warm (because the room is too warm, or their bedding is too warm) they can overheat.
- Don't put blankets over their head.
- Sleep sacks need to be the right size for the weight of your baby, and the right thickness (or tog rating) for the temperature of your room.
- Don't use a sleep sack *and* a blanket at the same time.
- You should not use nests or pods for baby to sleep in, or 'bumpers' to go around cots. These are not safe, as they can reduce the amount of oxygen around baby's face.
- Car seats and baby bouncers are also not safe for baby to sleep in for a long time. This is because they can have difficulty breathing. If baby falls asleep on a short car journey that's OK, but longer journeys should be split up.

The risk of sudden infant death syndrome is much higher if you fall asleep with baby on a sofa or armchair. One reason for this is because these seats are softer and the baby might end up in a position where they can't breathe. Also, it isn't safe for you to fall asleep with baby in a sling or carrier (see pages 298–299 for more information).

! It is really dangerous to fall asleep with baby when you are on a sofa or armchair.

? When is it unsafe to co-sleep?

- You should **never** co-sleep on a sofa or armchair, or if your mattress isn't firm.
- If anyone in the bed:

  - has drunk alcohol
  - smokes cigarettes
  - takes drugs or medication that makes them sleepy.
- If you:
  - are extremely tired or unwell.
- If your baby:
  - was born early (prematurely), before they were 37 weeks
  - was a low birthweight baby, below 5.5 lb or 2.5 kg when they were born
  - has a fever or is unwell.

You can watch a video about safer co-sleeping here:

Normal baby communication: my baby cries a lot

Babies' crying is designed to be like a very loud alarm, because human babies are not able to look after themselves.

Also, babies cry for lots of different reasons. They could be hungry, have a wet or dirty nappy, have wind (needing to burp), be too hot or too cold, feel overstimulated (which can be because of lots of visitors) or just need a cuddle.

You may also find that there is a time of day when your baby tends to be upset and can't be soothed when crying a lot.

After eight weeks, babies tend to cry less, so this stage won't last forever, even if it feels never ending.

You can watch an Autistic NICU (neonatal intensive care unit) nurse talk about why babies cry here:

Babies crying – especially with sleep deprivation happening for you too – can be a lot for Autistic parents, especially if you already struggle with being sensitive to sounds.

What Autistic people said... about their baby crying

- It was important to use things to help them be less dysregulated, like earplugs or noise cancelling headphones. This cut down the noise, but they could usually still hear the baby enough to know they were safe.
- If it got overwhelming, they put the baby down (somewhere safe) and had a break for a few minutes to calm down. This could include being in a dark and quiet room, dancing to a favourite song, having a shower or crying themselves.
- When trying to work out baby's needs, it could be helpful to develop a go-to list that they ran through until the baby was calm, such as checking if they were hungry, had a dirty nappy, were tired and needed to be soothed to sleep, or just wanted to be held.
- Some who usually find loud noises difficult felt a rush of empathy for their baby instead of the pain that other loud noises caused.

You can watch an Autistic parent talk about their experience of their baby crying here:

Soothing a crying baby

There are quite a few ways to soothe a crying baby. You may find some work for your baby, and others don't. Don't feel that you need to use things that don't work – even if others tell you they should.

Tool: My baby is crying – what should I try to soothe them?

This is a basic list that you might want to update when you know more about your baby's needs.

- Check their basic needs are met:
  - Do they have a wet or dirty nappy?
  - If they've just had a feed, do they need winding?
  - Are they hungry? How long ago did they last feed?
- The boob – if you're breastfeeding, let your baby suckle (even if they've recently eaten).
- Hold your baby (or use a carrier or sling) and try one or more of these:
  - Move your body – rock, sway, walk, pace.
  - Talk to them, hum or sing.
  - Stroke their back firmly, or massage them gently and firmly.
- Distract them:
  - Give them something to look at or listen to.
  - Take them for a walk in their pram or sling.
  - Put them in their pram and rock the pram backwards and forwards.
  - Take them for a drive (but newborns can only stay in a car seat for 30 minutes).

Colic

Colic is the name for when a baby **regularly** cries excessively – this can sometimes be for hours at a time.

We don't know why some babies get colic. All you can do at the time they are inconsolable is try to comfort them. You should also speak to your health professional to get reassurance that it is colic and not something else.

It is very normal for parents of babies with colic to feel upset, overwhelmed and frustrated. If the crying gets too much for you, put baby down somewhere safe and go to another room to decompress for a few minutes. You could also see if somebody else could take a shift with the baby to give you a longer break.

If your baby doesn't usually cry constantly and starts doing this suddenly, they might be poorly. You should seek medical attention.

Normal baby feeding patterns

These days, instead of feeding babies on a set schedule, it is recommended that parents look out for hunger cues and feed their baby 'on demand'. This is sometimes called 'responsive feeding'.

What are the signs my baby may be hungry?

When your baby is hungry, they will do things like:

- sucking their fists
- licking their lips
- wriggling around and opening their mouth.

If you miss these signs, your baby might start to cry. It can be harder to get a baby to feed when they're crying, so it's good to look out for the early signs and to offer them a feed then.

When your baby is first born, their tummy is the size of a marble or a cherry. This means that they can only take a tiny amount of milk before they are full. Because babies need lots of energy to grow, this means they will feed very often in the first few weeks: 12 times a day is perfectly normal.

They can also do something called 'cluster feeding', when they have lots of feeds one after another. You may find that baby has times of day when they feed a lot.

If you are breastfeeding, when babies are cluster feeding, you (or those around you) may think that you are not producing enough milk. However, your body will make milk in response to how often the baby feeds.

As baby's tummy grows, there may be longer gaps between feeds. But babies have regular developmental leaps and growth spurts, and will often feed more before and during these. Baby may also breastfeed for comfort and reassurance, not just because they are hungry, latching onto the breast but not always sucking. It's also normal for babies to pause during feeds.

This is normal, as long as:

- you hear swallowing when baby is feeding
- baby is putting on weight when they get weighed
- baby is producing enough wet and dirty nappies (from day 5 onwards, at least six wet nappies and at least two dirty nappies a day – ask your midwife if you're unsure)
- baby is having some periods of settled time
- your nipples are not sore.

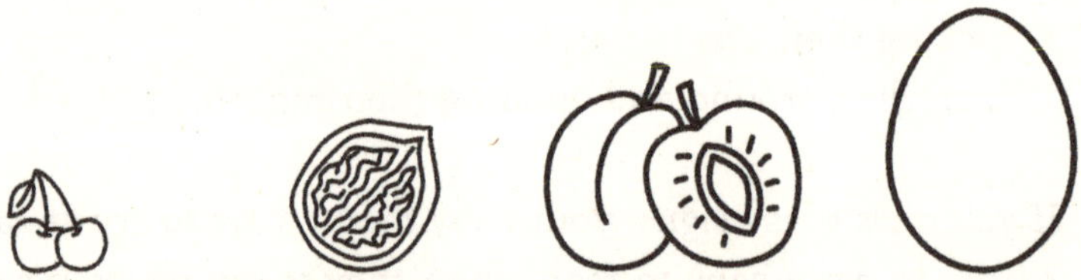

Day 1	**Day 3**	**One week**	**One month**
Size of a cherry	Size of a walnut	Size of an apricot	Size of a large egg
about 6 ml	about 27 ml	45–60 ml	80–150 ml

An illustration of a newborn's stomach size

Breastmilk is meant to be digested quickly, so baby is ready for the next feed sooner than with infant formula. If you are formula feeding, there may be longer gaps between feeds because babies take longer to digest infant formula.

! Newborn babies have very small tummies, so it's normal for them to need to feed about 12 times a day.

Safe ways to feed your baby

For the first six months of your baby's life, they get **all** of the nutrition they need from human milk or infant formula. They do not need any other food or drink. This means babies aged up to six months **do not** need:

- water
- baby tea
- baby rice
- any food at all.

There are **only three** safe types of milk to feed to your new baby:

- your own breastmilk
- screened donor breastmilk
- infant formula (also known as a 'breastmilk substitute').

! Babies only need breastmilk or infant formula until they are six months old.

Let's look at each of these one at a time, to understand the basics.

Breastfeeding

Breastmilk is clever stuff; it helps to protect babies from tummy, chest and ear infections. Breastfed babies are also less likely to have asthma and allergies.

Breastfeeding also reduces the risk of breast and ovarian cancer in the parent who breastfeeds.

But it can be difficult to breastfeed, and parents are not often told in advance that breastfeeding can be challenging.

You can watch an Autistic parent talk about the things she wishes she had been told about breastfeeding here:

What happens to the parent when you breastfeed?

Breastmilk is produced in grape-like clusters of cells (called alveoli). The milk then travels along the milk ducts to the nipple.

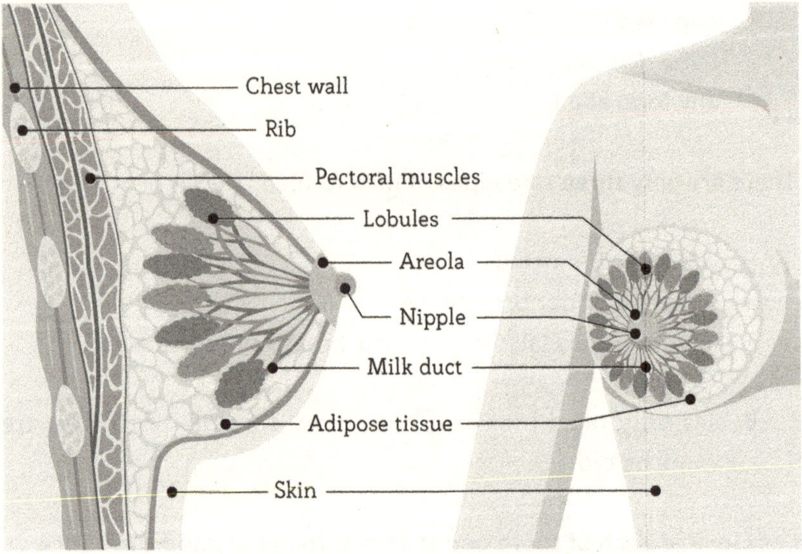

A drawing of female breast anatomy

When your baby sucks on the nipple, hormones are released which help your breasts produce milk and move it to the nipple.

Many parents can feel or sense when their body starts to move milk to the nipple. This is called the milk let-down reflex.

What Autistic people said... about the milk let-down reflex

- It could feel weird or uncomfortable.
- Some people hated the sensation of the milk let-down reflex.
- Some people didn't feel it at all (because they had low interoception).
- Milk coming out before the baby was latched could feel uncomfortable on their skin.

- The oxytocin that came with a let-down could feel calming.

Whilst your body does some of the work of making milk by itself, getting the milk from the breast into baby is a skill. This means it often takes time and practice for both the baby and you to work out how to breastfeed.

How do I get baby to breastfeed?

It's known as 'latching on' when baby suckles. New babies can find it hard to suckle in the way that lets the milk flow, so it's a learning experience for baby as well as you.

What is a good 'latch' when breastfeeding?

Not every latch will be 'good'.

By 'good' I mean it is comfortable for you, doesn't cause you pain and – very importantly – allows baby to get the milk.

Some signs of a good latch are:

- baby's head should be straight, not turned to the side, with baby's chest and stomach resting against your body
- baby's chin should touch your breast
- baby's mouth should be wide open and have most of your areola (the darker bit around the nipple) in their mouth, not just your nipple
- baby's nose should be clear of the breast.

You can see a 'Start for Life' guide to baby latching on with pictures here:

When you are in a good position and can comfortably hold baby, this can help both of you get used to breastfeeding. This can also take some practice.

The traditional way that you often see pictured is the 'cradle', with baby held across your body in your arms.

There are lots of other ways to hold baby when you feed, including 'laid back', where you recline with baby lying on your tummy, a 'rugby' or 'football' hold, where baby's body goes around the side of your body, and lying on your side with baby lying beside you.

It is very difficult to describe positioning in writing, but there are lots of guides available online. The most important thing is that you are comfortable and baby is able to feed well.

You can watch an Autistic maternity support worker talk about how to position your baby here:

If you struggle with breastfeeding, and especially knowing if you and baby have got a good latch, you are definitely not alone.

Another thing that can be difficult for Autistic parents is the sensory side of breastfeeding.

You can watch an Autistic antenatal educator talk about sensory issues when breastfeeding here:

What Autistic people said... about the sensory side of breastfeeding

- Having baby's body close to theirs for so long could be really nice for some.
- It could also help them to self-regulate when feeling overwhelmed.
- For others, baby being close for so much time was a

lot (and sometimes too much), as baby was warm and moving.

- Some people talked about the intensity of breastfeeding, such as feeling 'touched out', and needed breaks away from baby.
- Baby sucking could be a funny sensation and noise.
- Some people found breastfeeding painful.
- Distraction, like playing on their phone, helped people to cope with difficult sensory parts of breastfeeding.

A few days after birth, you may notice that your breastmilk starts to change. This is the change from the first type of milk (colostrum) to breastmilk.

You can watch an Autistic lactation consultant talk about the change from colostrum to breastmilk here:

You can watch an Autistic parent talk about their breastfeeding experiences here:

Getting help with breastfeeding

There are lots of common issues that come up about feeding babies. We'll talk about them later in the chapter. Here we'll think specifically about getting help with breastfeeding.

The help available with feeding your baby will vary from country to country, and may even be different in different areas of a country. But there should always be some support available.

Who can help me with breastfeeding?

Role	Training in breastfeeding
Breastfeeding peer supporter	Usually volunteers with experience of breastfeeding their own child, and some training.
Breastfeeding counsellor	Like peer supporters, but have had more training.
Registered health professionals, e.g. midwife, health visitor/public health nurse, doctor/paediatrician	There is no standardized in-depth training in supporting breastfeeding for these health professionals. They may have had *less* breastfeeding training than a peer supporter.
Lactation consultant (sometimes called IBCLC, or International Board Certified Lactation Consultant)	Has undergone the most extensive breastfeeding training. Can also be a midwife, doctor or nurse, but has a separate qualification.

When getting help in person, the breastfeeding supporter shouldn't be touching your breast or the back of baby's head. They should also always ask your permission before touching you.

Many countries will have a breastfeeding telephone helpline. Also, there are large numbers of Facebook breastfeeding support groups, where parents provide support to each other (including in the middle of the night!).

Script: How to ask for help with breastfeeding

In a healthcare consultation, with a midwife or doctor, you may need to be very quick and to the point.

- 'I'm Autistic, so that means I really don't want you to touch me.'
- 'If you want to touch me, please give me enough time to decide and tell you if I agree or not.'
- 'I'm breastfeeding and I'm finding (thing) difficult. Do you have any advice?'
- 'I'm breastfeeding and...

- I'm not sure if our latch is right - would you be able to watch a feed?'
- I don't know if I might have damage to my nipple - could you have a look?'
- I think I could have mastitis (tell them your symptoms).'
- I'm worried that baby isn't getting enough milk - they've had (number) of wet nappies, and (number) of dirty nappies yesterday.'
- I'm not feeling very confident. Do you know if there are any breastfeeding support groups locally?'

In a breastfeeding support group, it's a bit different. People will often be sat in a rough circle, and there may be some babies in the middle on the floor. Older children may be playing in other parts of the room. Sometimes there are drinks and biscuits.

You could start by asking the person closest to you, or who you see looking at you:

- 'Could you point out the peer supporters to me? I could do with some help with feeding' (hopefully they would then introduce you to a peer supporter).
- 'Do you know if a midwife or health professional comes to the group?'

It is common to feel anxious about seeking help with breastfeeding, and might be even more anxiety-inducing for some Autistic people. It may help you to know that peer supporters, breastfeeding counsellors and lactation consultants spend nearly all of their time supporting breastfeeding.

You can watch an Autistic midwife talk about contacting your midwife for any worries about you or baby here:

Also, when it comes to peer supporters, many start being a breastfeeding supporter because they didn't get enough help with their baby and they want to make sure others don't have that negative experience.

Health professionals such as midwives, health visitors and doctors may know a lot about supporting breastfeeding, but they might not. If you still feel unsure after speaking to one of them, you might want to get a second opinion.

What Autistic people said... about breastfeeding support

- Some people had really good experiences, which they said helped them to keep breastfeeding.
- Sometimes the support given didn't actually help with breastfeeding.
- Some people were told conflicting (different) things, which they found unhelpful.
- Some people felt like they weren't listened to.
- Breastfeeding groups could be a lot of sensory input all at once.

Expressing your breastmilk

Feeding your own breastmilk includes feeding baby directly from your chest and expressing (sometimes called 'pumping') your milk. Some people express so that others can feed their baby or because their baby is unable to directly breastfeed, but some Autistic people choose to express all of the time, as they prefer it over feeding directly from the chest. Expressing can be done by hand or using a pump.

You can watch an Autistic parent talk about their experiences of expressing here:

Let's talk about hand expressing first. There is no single 'right' way to hand express, it's whatever feels most comfortable to you whilst producing milk. It should not be painful.

How do I express my breastmilk by hand?

- Make the space around you as relaxed as you can, to help the milk come out.
- Wash your hands.
- If you want to save the milk for your baby, you must use a sterilized container to collect the milk.
- **Optional step:** If your milk doesn't come out easily, you can do things to help, such as:
  - gently massaging your breast, from the wall of your chest to your nipple
  - using a warm towel on your breast
  - having a warm shower or bath.
- Put **gentle** pressure on your milk ducts – they're about an inch behind your areola (the dark bit around your nipple). You could try to:
  - cup your breast with one hand and make a C shape with the thumb and fingers of the other hand
  - use both hands around one breast with both thumbs pointing up.
- Gently, using light pressure, press your hands towards your chest wall to squeeze and release in a rhythm similar to a baby feeding from the breast. Your fingers should stay in the same place on the breast.
- You should hopefully start to see some milk – this can either be droplets on the nipple, a spray of milk or a trickle – all are normal.
- If you don't see any drops of milk, try moving your hand or hands slightly closer to the nipple or further away from the nipple, but still keep your hand off the nipple.
- When the milk flow slows down, rotate the position of your hand (not whilst squeezing the breast) so that you will be releasing milk from another milk duct. You can

express all around your breast to ensure all milk ducts get emptied.

- When you've finished, you can express from the other breast.
- If you are trying to build your supply, you can express all around one breast, and then the other, and repeat until the milk stops flowing.

You can watch an Autistic midwifery support worker talk about how to hand express here:

If you still aren't sure, or you've tried this and don't think it's working, you can ask your midwife or another breastfeeding supporter for help. They can help you work out where your milk ducts are (they may need to touch you to do this, or you can ask them to describe it to you), and to check your technique.

Breast pumps

Breast pumps should not be used at all whilst you are pregnant.

If your health professional thinks that you may have a low milk supply, they may suggest that as well as letting baby feed from the breast, you also use a breast pump between feeds to try to increase your supply. This is because your body will make as much milk as is needed (it's possible to breastfeed twins and even to 'tandem feed' an older infant and a new baby).

You may be able to borrow or rent a breast pump from your local breastfeeding support group or maternity unit; your midwife will usually know if there is a local scheme.

Breast pumps come in two varieties: manual, where you need to squeeze the pump using your hand; or electric, which does the squeezing for you. If you use a pump, rather than your hands, to express milk you plan to feed to your baby, you need to make sure the pump is sterilized.

If you have a sick or premature baby, you need to sterilize it every time you pump. Otherwise, you can store all of the equipment in a sealed clean container in the fridge and wash and sterilize it once a day.

We talk about different ways to sterilize things later in the chapter.

Regardless of the type of pump you use, it's important that it fits your nipple. The 'funnel' or 'flange' is the part that goes over your nipple, and it should be snug but not tight. When you buy a pump, they often include multiple sizes of funnels. Like hand expressing, it shouldn't hurt, so if it hurts, you should ask for advice from somebody knowledgeable about breastfeeding.

Electric pumps can often be set to different strengths, and it is recommended to use a lower setting when you start, or it can be painful (and may damage your nipple).

What Autistic people said... about expressing breastmilk

- More Autistic parents expressed most of the time than non-Autistic parents. This means it was better for them than feeding from the breast.
- Some could find it unpleasant to express, because of the noise or the suction feeling.

If you want to try expressing with a pump, it's absolutely OK to use whatever things help to distract you from the noise and sensation. Also, trying a range of pumps may help you to find the most tolerable pump.

How to store expressed milk

After you have expressed, you can save the milk for your baby as long as it is in a sterilized sealed container. You can keep a sterilized container in the fridge and add expressed milk to this throughout the day. When storing milk, put the date on the container so you know when it was expressed.

Breastmilk should not be stored in the door of a fridge, as the temperature changes there each time the door is opened, and it could go off more quickly. The temperature of the place the milk is stored impacts how long it is safe to keep:

Location	Time limit
Room temperature (unless the room is very hot)	6 hours
Fridge (above 4 °C or 39 °F)	3 days
Fridge (below 4 °C or 39 °F)	8 days
Freezer (below -18 °C or 0 °F)	6 months

If you freeze breastmilk, you should defrost it in the fridge, and it can take up to 12 hours to defrost. If you need the milk to defrost more quickly, you can run it under warm water from a tap. Never use boiling water or a microwave to defrost breastmilk.

Once you start feeding expressed breastmilk to your baby, it should be used within one to two hours and then any milk left should be thrown away.

You can feed expressed milk to baby in a bottle, or if you have training from a health professional you can use a cup or syringe. The bottle or other feeding equipment used to feed baby also needs to be washed and sterilized after every use. You can read more about using a bottle to feed baby later in the chapter.

If you find that you have more breastmilk than you need, you may be able to donate to your local donor human milk bank. They will often ask you to complete some questions about your health and you may need to have a blood test to check for any diseases.

You can watch an Autistic midwifery support worker talk about safely storing expressed breastmilk here:

Sterilizing infant feeding equipment

If you are using any 'equipment' when feeding your baby, it will need to be washed **and** sterilized. Examples of equipment include:

- nipple shields
- breast pumps to express

- bottles, including teat, ring, cap and other parts of the bottle that you use to feed expressed breastmilk or formula.

There are several different ways to sterilize your feeding equipment.

How can I sterilize my feeding equipment?

You should always wash your feeding equipment before sterilizing, to get rid of as much of the old milk as possible.

Always make sure you follow the manufacturer's instructions with sterilizing solutions, steamers and UV (ultraviolet) sterilizers.

There are five main types of sterilizing:

- cold water – you buy liquid or tablets that you put into a container of cold water
- steam
- boiling in a pan – this is harshest on the bottles and teats, so it's important to check them for damage
- microwave
- UV.

You can watch an Autistic midwife and lactation consultant talk about sterilizing feeding equipment here:

Donor human milk

Donor breastmilk may be a new concept to many people reading this book. Historically this would be called having a 'wet nurse'. If you are unable or do not want to breastfeed, you may wish to try to access donor breastmilk to get some of the benefits of breastfeeding.

This can happen in two ways, first from a human milk bank. These are often found at hospitals, and they will generally screen the milk for diseases. Because human milk banks often don't receive enough milk for all babies, it is often reserved for premature or sick babies.

Second, you may be able to get donor milk directly from another person who has recently had a baby. This is usually arranged through social media, including via the organization Human Milk 4 Human Babies, or parent to parent, when a breastfeeding parent has an over-supply of milk.

This isn't generally recommended by health services, because the safety of the milk can't be guaranteed if it is accessed outside of a milk bank. For example, the milk may not have been stored in a way to prevent bacteria from growing. It also won't have been screened. If you ever have any concerns about the safety of donor milk given to you directly by another parent, speak to a health professional before using it.

Infant formula

There is an overwhelming amount of choice when it comes to buying things related to formula feeding, but you really don't need to buy everything available.

? What do I need to formula feed my baby?

- Several bottles, including the ring and cap:
  - Bottles come in different sizes, but any size is fine for a newborn – older babies will need bigger bottles.
  - Remember you'll need to sterilize the bottles after each use.
- Teats:
  - Teats have different 'flow rates', which means how much milk comes out. For new babies, slow flow is usually a good choice.
  - There are different shapes of teats. There is no evidence that one shape is better than another... although your baby may have a preference.
- A bottle brush to be used only for washing the bottles and teats.
- Sterilizing equipment.
- Infant formula – either powdered or ready to feed liquid (see below).

Infant formula most commonly comes as tubs of powder that are made into liquid milk with water.

? How do I choose the right infant formula for my baby?

- There are **a lot** of different products on sale.
- **But** this is a marketing strategy; infant formula is highly regulated so the ingredients will be very, very similar, regardless of brand.
- The cheapest available will be almost identical to the most expensive.
- Formula-fed babies **only need** first infant formula, which they can drink until they are 12 months of age, and you can then introduce other forms of milk, like cow's milk or soya.

! Formula-fed babies only need first infant formula, and all brands will be very similar.

The World Health Organization says that the water used should be boiled in a kettle and used to make up the milk when it is between 70 °C and 100 °C (158–212 °F).

Using water that is this temperature is important because powdered formula can contain bacteria that can make babies very poorly (and in rare cases there have been deaths from this), and water that is at least 70 °C kills those bacteria.

The advice to parents in some countries follows the 70 °C rule, but this is not used in all countries. My personal recommendation is to follow the 70 °C rule. It's really important to then cool the milk to drinking temperature, such as by putting the cap on the bottle and holding it under cool running water.

In many countries, parents are able to buy infant formula preparation machines. There are two major safety concerns with these machines:

1. The water may not reach 70 °C, or may not stay at 70 °C for long enough to kill any bacteria in the formula.

2. The inside of the machines may hold bacteria.

When making a bottle of formula, use a kettle to heat the water, as infant formula preparation machines may be unsafe.

How do I prepare a bottle of infant formula?

Making up powdered formula involves lots of steps to reduce the risk of baby becoming poorly.

I recommend following the UK NHS guidance:

You can see the NHS advice on making a bottle here:

You can also watch an Autistic midwife and lactation consultant talk about how to make up a bottle of formula here:

What Autistic people said... about making bottles of formula

- Most people found it easy to understand the instructions on the formula tub.
- Some people were anxious about making formula safely.
- Some people found the advice they were given and instructions confusing.
- Not knowing when baby would next want a feed could make it difficult to prepare formula at the right time.
- Needing to have sterilized bottles ready could feel overwhelming.

It is also possible in some countries, like the UK, to buy bottles of ready-to-drink infant formula that are sterile. This is usually much more expensive than using powdered formula, but can be easier when taking baby out and about, when you may not have access to a kettle.

How do I bottle feed my baby?

It's really important to **never** prop a bottle up so baby can feed themselves. If the bottle is propped up, they can choke on the milk.

- Hold your baby semi-upright and support their head.
- Keep the bottle almost horizontal – this reduces the amount of air they swallow.
- Let them have regular breaks. Watch for splayed fingers; this is a sign your baby needs a pause.
- Let your baby decide when they've had enough – don't worry if they don't take a whole bottle.
- After they've eaten, hold them upright and rub or pat their back gently so they can burp out any wind.
- Thow away any leftover formula within an hour of baby starting the feed – this is very important because baby's saliva means that bacteria will grow more quickly in formula that they've been eating.

Baby might be a little bit sick after feeds – this is called reflux.

If they are sick after feeds a lot, check that you are following the advice above – especially not making them drink more than they want. If you are worried about them being sick, they are not having lots of wet and dirty nappies or anything else, ask your health professional.

When bottle feeding, never ever prop a bottle up for baby to drink alone. Also, throw away any left-over formula within an hour of starting the feed – both of these are very important for your baby's safety.

It's also important to remember that you'll need to wash and sterilize baby's bottles and any other feeding equipment every time they use them. The UK NHS recommend this is done until baby is 12 months old. This is because bacteria can grow in the milk that's left inside the teat and bottle. We talked about sterilizing earlier in the chapter.

! It's important to wash and sterilize baby's bottles and other feeding equipment after every feed.

Common worries

It's very normal for parents to worry about if feeding is going well.

Below we have some answers to common concerns that Autistic parents have about crying, sleep and feeding.

What Autistic people said... about their feeding worries

Worry	Answer
They're feeding all of the time; I'm exhausted	This is normal in the first few months. Try to: • rest when you can • take any help you can from others • look at Chapter 13, which focuses on your mental health. It might help to know that it does get easier – some Autistic parents said 6 weeks was when it got easier for them. Also look out for the signs of infection – in any stitches, as well as your breasts, as Autistic people don't always notice these. You could also check your temperature, as a high or low temperature is also a sign of infection.
It hurts when I breastfeed	It's common to get a bit of pain when baby first latches on, but it should go quickly. If it carries on hurting, there may be an issue with baby's latch. Cracks or bleeding nipples are not normal. If you have pain, cracked or bleeding nipples, it would be a good idea to get advice from a health professional or breastfeeding supporter.

It doesn't hurt when I breastfeed, but my nipple is bleeding and doesn't look normal	Some Autistic people don't feel pain from a latch that isn't good. This means their nipples can get damaged. It's a good idea to get some help from a health professional or breastfeeding supporter to help you and baby get a better latch.
My baby is struggling to latch. I think they could have a tongue tie.	This is definitely the time to get some support from a health professional or breastfeeding supporter.
I'm worried my baby isn't getting enough milk, or baby isn't gaining enough weight	This is a common worry for parents. Signs that baby is getting enough milk include: • having at least six wet nappies per day from day 5 onwards • having at least two dirty nappies per day from day 5 onwards, with the poos at least the size of a £2 coin • being active and alert in between feeds. If you have any worries speak to your health professional.
My baby is being sick a lot after feeding (they have reflux)	This can be a sign they are having too much milk too quickly. If you don't think that's the case, speak to your health professional for advice.
I think I want to stop breastfeeding, but feel upset or guilty about this	Feeding is one aspect of looking after a baby, and if breastfeeding is not right for you that is OK. It's also common for parents to feel sad or guilty when this happens. It doesn't make it easier for you, but reaching out to other parents might help you feel less alone.
Breastfeeding feels awful, but I want to carry on	Check with a health professional or breastfeeding supporter to make sure baby's latch is as good as it can be. Try some other breastfeeding positions, to see if there is one that's better for you. Know that bonding with baby isn't impacted by you distracting yourself on your phone or by doing something else for distraction when feeding. Many Autistic parents used distraction to help them get through difficult feeds.

cont.

Worry	Answer
I'm being pressured to stop breastfeeding (or to continue breastfeeding)	Many parents have this issue. The way that baby is fed is primarily down to the birthing parent, and your wellbeing is very important. In Chapter 5 we talked about strategies to shut down people pressuring you to do things you don't want to do. This includes 'grey rocking', where you stop engaging with people and remove yourself from the situation.
I'm worried about breastfeeding outside of the home	This is a very common worry. In many countries you have the legal right to breastfeed in public spaces. You may feel safer if you check the law in your area. Lots of breastfeeding parents have their first feed at a breastfeeding support group and build their confidence up in these safe spaces first. Some areas have programmes like 'breastfeeding welcome' where venues can sign up to say they especially welcome breastfeeding. You could ask about this or places parents in your area find comfortable to breastfeed in a local 'mums' Facebook group. Some parents find that using a cover or shawl helps them feel more comfortable. Others try to express milk to take with them in a bottle, but this is extra work.

You can watch an Autistic midwifery support worker talk about common breastfeeding issues here:

Weaning

Your baby does not need anything other than breastmilk or infant formula until they are six months old. After this, you can gradually start to introduce food.

But this doesn't mean that others won't try to encourage you to feed them other drinks and food sooner.

Script: What to say to people who want you to wean your baby earlier than recommended

- 'Thank you, I've spoken to the (midwife, doctor, etc.) and they have said not to until baby is six months old.'
- 'We've decided to follow the World Health Organization guidance. They've reviewed all of the evidence and decided what is safest.'
- 'No, baby doesn't need anything other than breastmilk/ formula.'

An Autistic midwife's top tips... on sleep, crying and feeding

By Rebecca Warboys, RM, IBCLC

- If you are wide awake and happy to cuddle your baby when they sleep, then do! This is brilliant for their brain development and for your bond with baby.
- If you are worried your room is warmer than 20 °C, keep your blinds or windows closed in the day. You can open the window, but do not put baby near a draught.
- If you're breastfeeding and don't have a good latch this impacts on how much milk is let down. This is because a good latch stimulates the nerves to make milk and to give a milk let-down.
- A shallow latch may mean baby takes longer to gain weight, longer to feed, wants to feed even more often, is not making enough wet and dirty nappies, seems more stressed or actually can be extra sleepy as they are not getting enough calories. Your nipples may also feel sore. Getting your latch checked as soon as possible if you are worried is a good idea.
- During hand expressing, if you are not seeing any milk/ colostrum coming out then make sure your thumb and fingers meet behind the nipple (where the milk ducts are), and not to the side.

- Babies can often cluster feed from the late afternoon/early evening and do so for several hours before settling for their first bedtime sleep. This is because the volume of milk is less on an evening but the percentage of fats in it is greater. It may feel like your breasts do not have enough milk but it's normal for them to feel softer at this time. Lots of side switching and knowing this is normal and will help increase your supply can help.
- Store breastmilk in a variety of volumes to make it easier to defrost and use what you need to have less wasted: for example, 15, 30 and 60 ml volumes.
- You should feed responsively even when formula feeding. This means just feeding when your baby shows feeding cues and feeding only as much as they want, not trying to encourage them to finish a bottle.
- Always have a change of clothes in the size baby needs (vest and sleepsuit) in your changing bag. Sometimes nappies can leak or baby may vomit, and you may need to change their clothes when out and about.

Conclusion

You've made it to the end of another chapter! We've covered a lot of different things you might experience in new parenting – including sleep, crying and a lot of information about the different ways you can feed baby. Overall, the most important thing is that you and baby are well and as comfortable as you can be. Next, we'll talk about other things it might be helpful to know about looking after a brand-new baby, although it's OK for you to go to whatever section you like.

CHAPTER 12

Caring For Your New Baby

CONTENTS

Introduction

In the previous chapter we thought about feeding your baby. Here we think about lots of other things you'll do when you're caring for your new baby.

We start off thinking about how to pick up your baby and hold them. This includes thinking about using carriers and slings, so you can go 'hands free'.

Next, we think about their poos and changing nappies and clothes, and bathing your baby.

Towards the end of the chapter we think about Autistic parenting styles, and how they might be different to what non-Autistic parents do, but that they are absolutely fine.

Last, we talk about social work assessments. Just because you are Autistic doesn't mean you need or should have an assessment, but this information is here so you know about them if it comes up.

There are a lot of new things for you to learn about, but don't worry – you'll get the hang of it soon, and if anything is worrying you or too difficult, you can look at the UK NHS website (www.nhs.uk) for more information, and if you still aren't sure, ask your health professional for advice.

! If you aren't sure about any part of looking after your baby, the UK NHS website is a good source of detailed information and videos. If you still aren't sure, ask your health professional.

Holding and carrying your baby

Caring for a new baby can feel very daunting, as they are so small and fragile.

It's also common for new babies to stay 'scrunched' in a foetal position for a month or two after birth. This is because they've been curled up in the womb and it takes time for them to stretch out.

Many people are worried about holding their new baby, and picking them up can be a particular worry.

? How do I safely hold a newborn baby?

The most important thing to remember is you must always support a newborn baby's head and neck. You'll need to keep on doing this until they can control their own head, which usually happens around four months of age.

- Slide one hand under baby's head and neck, making sure you only touch their 'soft spots' gently (see below).
- Slide your other hand under their bottom.
- When you feel that you have them securely in your hands, bring them close to your body.
- Do not let their head flop from side to side or front to back.

Babies need their head and neck to be supported **all of the time** (if they are not lying down) until they are about four months old.

It's also important to always be gentle when touching your baby's 'soft spots' on their head.

What is a 'soft spot' on my baby's head?

Babies have two 'soft spots' on their head. They are completely normal, and are where there are gaps in the bones of the skull.

The soft spot at the front is bigger than the one at the back.

Over time the soft spots will close up, but they are needed for human babies:

- to make vaginal birth possible – the bones of the skull can overlap, making the head smaller during birth
- to allow for lots of brain growth in the first 12–18 months after birth.

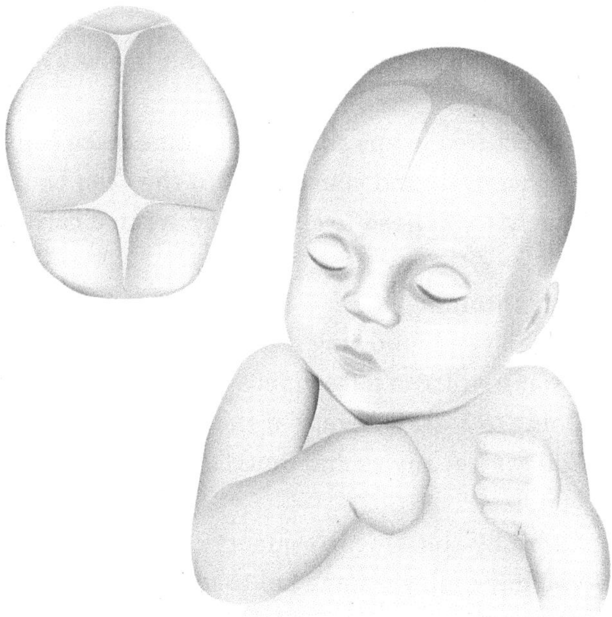

A drawing of soft spots on a baby's head

Using baby carriers and slings

In many cultures, 'wearing' babies with fabric to attach them to the parent's body is normal.

Before birth, your baby was used to being carried around in your body, hearing lots of noise and feeling the comforting beat of your heart. This means that being away from you can be frightening for them.

Wearing baby is also sometimes called 'kangaroo care'. It involves keeping your baby in a wrap, carrier or sling against your chest. This can help them feel more comfortable. It also allows you to hold the baby and keep your hands free to do other things.

These days you can buy a range of baby carriers – which tend to be structured – and 'slings', which are less structured pieces of fabric.

How do I find the right carrier or sling for me and my baby?

- Not all carriers or slings are safe to use with a newborn baby.
- More structured baby carriers might be less comfortable for you, as there are fixed straps (a bit like wearing a rucksack).
- Less structured wraps and slings can be more comfortable as they wrap around your body, but they can be harder to use safely – you need to check they are tied correctly each time.
- I highly recommend:
  - Reading and following the manufacturers' instructions – some will also have videos available.
  - Going to a 'sling library' if there is one in your area. You can get advice and rent a carrier or sling to see if you like it.
  - Carefully checking the quality of any slings or wraps you buy online – some fail to meet safety standards.

There are some risks to using a sling; some babies have been injured or died. This is because fabric from the sling or parents' clothes can cover the nose and mouth and young babies can't move their head out of the way, or because they have slipped and fallen out.

How do I safely use a sling or carrier?

The UK Sling Consortium has a 'T.I.C.K.S. rule for safe babywearing':

- (Slings should be)
  - Tight
- (Babies should be)
  - In view at all times
  - Close enough to kiss
  - Keep chin off the chest
  - Supported back.

You can read more about each of the five points here: https://babyslingsafety.co.uk/ticks.pdf

Wearing your baby in a sling or carrier can be really good for you both, but it is important to do it safely – remember T.I.C.K.S and don't go to sleep wearing baby in a sling.

What Autistic people said... about using carriers and slings

- There was some 'trial and error' trying to find the best carrier or sling.
- Some people preferred to have several options, or to change the type of carrier or sling as the baby grew.
- Going to a sling library helped some to find slings that met their needs, and to be confident that they were using them safely.

- Feeling the weight of baby in a sling could be regulating for some.
- Keeping baby this close helped the parent to learn their baby's cues.

Baby poo

If this is your first baby, you might be surprised at what their dirty nappies look like.

Is my baby's poo normal?

Baby poo changes a lot in the first week, as your baby has been producing a type of poo in the womb. This is called meconium.

- On the first two days, their poo can be very dark greenish-black, and sticky.
- On days 3–4, their poo looks lighter and more green or brown in colour.
- On days 5–6 it looks mustard yellow in colour and is like a liquidy paste if you are breastfeeding. If you are formula feeding, it may be firmer and darker brown.

From day 5, it's normal for baby to have at least two poos a day that are the size of a £2 coin (about an inch or 2.5 cm around). Some babies will poo a lot more.

The amount of poos a baby does might be less after around six weeks, and will go down to around two a day by the time they are 12 months old.

If your baby hasn't pooed in the last 24-48 hours or if you have any worries, ask your health professional.

! If your baby hasn't pooed for 24–48 hours ask your midwife or health professional. This can be a sign they aren't getting enough milk.

You can watch an Autistic maternity support worker talk about changes in baby's poo here:

The NCT have a written guide with pictures of normal baby poo – you can see it here:

Changing nappies

It's important to change your baby's nappy as soon as they pee or poo. For young babies this can mean at least 10–12 nappy changes a day.

If you don't change their wet and dirty nappies, they can get sore skin or nappy rash.

What is nappy rash?

Nappy rash can be caused by:

- wee or poo being in contact with baby's skin
- not cleaning the nappy area or changing the nappy often enough
- wipes or soap irritating the skin – using plain water with cotton wool pads, or wipes which are 99 per cent water, is best.

Nappy rash is when the skin surface starts to break down, and the skin looks red and sore. It can feel hot to touch. If nappy rash is severe, your baby may be uncomfortable and distressed. If this happens, speak to your health professional or a pharmacist to get some nappy rash cream.

! If your baby's nappy rash is making them uncomfortable, speak to a health professional or pharmacist to get some cream to treat it.

There are lots of things to think about and remember when changing a nappy.

? How can I prevent nappy rash?

- Change nappies as soon as they are wet or dirty.
- Clean the whole area with water or fragrance-free or alcohol-free baby wipes that are at least 99 per cent water.
- When cleaning, wipe from front to back.
- When you bathe your baby, leave them without a nappy for a while (lying on a towel in case they go to the toilet) so they get some fresh air.

One of the most important things is to make sure baby can't hurt themselves if they roll off the changing mat or table. This means keeping yourself between them and the edge of the changing surface (and the floor) at all times. Just because you haven't seen baby roll over yet, you still **always** need to be careful. This is because babies can accidentally put themselves on their side and can then fall on the floor and fracture bones. It only takes a second.

Once you get used to it, changing nappies will come easily for most people.

! When changing baby's nappy, make sure they can't roll or fall off a high surface; keep yourself between them and the edge of the changing table.

What Autistic people said... about changing nappies

- The sensory experience – especially the smell – could be a lot at first, but parents got used to this over time.
- Babies often showed that they needed a nappy change in the same way, but sometimes they didn't, and parents could feel bad that they didn't realize their baby was in a wet or dirty nappy.
- Some babies were sensitive to the chemicals in disposable wipes, or had sensitive skin.
- If their baby got nappy rash, some parents could feel very guilty, even when they treated it quickly.
- Many people used disposable nappies:
  - They were more convenient than cloth for many, but were more expensive overall.
- Some people preferred to use reusable cloth nappies:
  - Starting gradually and only using a few a day was a good way to 'ease in' if they'd already been using disposable nappies.
  - Nappy libraries were helpful to work out the best kind of nappy type for them.
  - Some people felt it was best to wash them soon after they were used or they could smell bad.
  - Keeping up with the washing could be overwhelming.
  - Using a nappy service could make it easier to keep up with the washing.
  - Buying cloth nappies second hand made the cost easier, and some people sold their cloth nappies when they had finished using them.

You can watch an NHS midwife talk about changing nappies at the bottom of this page:

Baby's clothes and temperature

In the early weeks, you'll find that you need quite a few changes of clothes. This is because baby may be sick on them or there may be an accident with their nappy.

At the same time, your baby will grow quickly, and will probably need bigger clothes within a few months. Many parents get baby clothes second hand to reduce the cost of this.

It's important to keep new babies warm enough, but not too hot. If babies get too hot, they are at risk of sudden infant death syndrome (SIDS). This is where they can be well and then quickly die (see Chapter 11, page 265 for more details about SIDS).

You can check baby's temperature by feeling their chest or the back ('nape') of their neck with your hand. If you'd find this difficult to judge, you can use a thermometer under their arm.

If baby looks sweaty or clammy, they are too hot and need to be wearing less clothes. If they feel cold when you touch their skin, they are too cold.

What types of clothes are best for baby?

It is good for baby's clothes to be:

- easy to take on and off – like:
  - romper suits that are made of stretchy material and do up down the front with poppers
  - tops with an 'envelope neck' which easily goes over their head
- soft and comfortable on baby's delicate skin
- made of natural fibres like cotton, especially if you're living in a hot climate.

Also, if you find some textures unpleasant, it makes sense to avoid those in baby's clothes if possible.

When you first start, it might feel stressful or difficult to get baby dressed, but you'll soon get used to it or find the clothes that are easiest for you to use.

How do I change my baby's clothes?

- Try to change them in a warm (not cold) room.
- Lie your baby down on a soft surface.
- Always be gentle; don't force the clothes on.
- Try not to let the clothes touch their face, as babies often cry when this happens.
- If you're using a romper with an opening down the front, open it up and lie baby on top of it, gently putting their arms and legs into the arm- and leg-holes. Then do up the poppers.
- If you're using a top that goes over their head, remember to support their head as you put it on.

You can watch a video about how to dress a newborn baby here:

Baby's first bath and skin care

You should wait until the cord (on baby's belly button) has dropped off before they have their first bath.

New babies' skin is very sensitive. This means they only need a bath two or three times a week.

The important bits of the baby to wash each day are their face, neck, hands, genitals and bottom.

Bathing your baby in the first few weeks is something many parents worry about. There are some important safety steps to consider.

Your baby doesn't need a full bath every day, but you should wash their hands, face, neck and nappy area every day.

? How can I safely bath my baby?

- Make sure the water isn't too hot. This means:
  - Mixing the water well with your hand so there are no hot patches **AND** checking the temperature is comfortable with your wrist or elbow.
  - If you struggle with telling temperatures, use a thermometer – the safe temperature for water is 37–38 °C (98–100 °F).
- You only need a small amount of water – around 8–10 cm (3–4 inches).
- Use plain water (no baby bath) – it's best for your baby's skin for the first month.
- You should hold the baby and not lie them down or prop them up in the bath.
- Never leave your baby alone in the bath, even for a second to answer the door or look after another child – always take your baby out of the bath first.

! You should **always** check the temperature of baby's bath water, **always** hold the baby in the bath, and **never** leave your baby alone in the bath, even for a second.

Young babies might be shocked by the temperature change of getting undressed and having a bath.

? How do I help baby enjoy baths?

- Bath your baby when they are awake and happy, not straight after a feed or when they're tired or hungry.
- Get everything ready before undressing baby.
- Make sure the room is warm enough (not cold).

You can watch a video from the UK NHS on how to bath your baby here:

Being an Autistic parent

You may have spent a lot of your life being told the way that you do things is wrong, and parenting is definitely very important, so it's natural to be a bit worried.

But I would try to encourage you to think about all of the positive connections you've made in your life, and to gain confidence that you already know your baby and they know you. The talking and moving you've been doing as they've been growing inside you mean that there is already a familiarity for the baby.

Also, the way that people raise their children is impacted by their life circumstances. This includes things like how much money they have, how safe and supportive the place they live in is, and how much support they have from their partner, family and friends.

There are also 'trends' in how people think it's best to raise a baby. Many of these come from new information (from research), which means that health professionals change the information given to parents. So, what your parents were told to do for the best for you is likely out of date in some ways now.

What this means is that there isn't a single 'right' way to parent your baby...even if some people tell you there is.

There is no single 'right' way to look after and connect with your baby.

The main things are to avoid harming yourself or your baby, and to keep the baby away from those who could harm them or you.

Doing things to attend to your own needs, like putting the baby down somewhere safe for a few minutes because their crying may otherwise push you into a meltdown or shutdown, **is completely OK.**

Putting your baby down somewhere safe and giving yourself a few minutes to re-regulate is always OK.

Some people also make a big deal about parents needing to keep eye contact with their baby. If this is painful for you, don't feel like you need to force it. Others may say that just because you are Autistic you aren't able to be a good parent – that's completely false.

Instead, you could think about if there is another way that is easy and comfortable for you to connect with them, which could be sharing a special interest. This could include doing an 'info dump' about a topic you enjoy talking about or showing them objects that you like (keeping them at a safe distance if they're breakable or could be dangerous for a tiny baby). This is because the baby will hear your voice and feel connected to you, even though they don't understand the words.

You could also think about whether there are any stims you could incorporate when caring for them. For example, if you find rocking soothing, could you put them in a sling or baby carrier whilst you rock? Does a particular song always calm you down when you sing it? If so, try singing it to them. Do you enjoy touching tactile surfaces? If yes, could your baby's clothing become something soothing for you to gently stroke?

Over time, you will get to know your child's needs, for example if one particular cry is because they are hungry or if they just want some company. You'll also find out the things that they enjoy you doing. In the early weeks and months, they may not have much of an attention span, so if something doesn't get a positive reaction, you could try again another day.

What Autistic people said... about negative reactions to them being a parent

- Many felt that they were watched or judged by others.
- Occasionally family members said that they should give their baby up for adoption or foster care, despite there being no concerns about the baby's health.
- Where parents had ended a relationship with a difficult or

abusive ex-partner, the ex-partner sometimes argued that they should have full-time custody because the birthing parent was Autistic.

- Getting support from domestic abuse organizations, free law centres or lawyers was important if any threats were made about having baby removed.

You can watch an Autistic social worker talk about Autistic parenting styles here:

Social work assessments

When you are pregnant, you have full rights over your child, but as soon as they are born this changes, and the child has their own rights. These rights will vary by country, but in general, children's rights are that they should be kept safe from harm and have their needs met.

Social workers can become involved with those who are pregnant or new parents either at the parent's request, or because a health professional has suggested it.

Tool: Should I ask for a social work assessment?

This is a really hard question to answer.

The first and most important question is:

- Do you feel like you're unable to look after the baby? For example, do you think you might harm yourself or the baby?

If yes, and you feel unsafe or very overwhelmed:

- It's important to seek help; this might initially be asking for more help from your partner (if you have one), friends and family.

- If that help isn't enough, it's important to speak to a health professional or to reach out to social work yourself.

If no, and you feel safe to look after the baby, I suggest that you make a list of pros and cons. These questions and ideas might help you:

- What are the things you are struggling with?
- What sort of help do you want or need?
- Can you look online (e.g. forums, Facebook mums' groups in your area) and see people's experiences of having social work involved – do they give the sorts of help you want?

If a health professional recommends you have a social work assessment, it doesn't automatically mean there are concerns about 'child protection'. By child protection, I include a risk of abuse (including from partners and other people you live with), or your ability to look after the child.

! Having a social work assessment doesn't mean there are concerns about abuse.

If you shared your Autism diagnosis with your maternity health professionals, they may automatically suggest you are seen by a social worker, even though there is no evidence that this is necessary.

Also, if your maternity health professional thought that you or your baby were being abused at home ('domestic abuse'), they **have** to refer you for an assessment. This includes things like being controlled by your partner, including financial control, or being emotionally, physically or sexually abused.

In each country there will be a list of things that midwives will automatically have to make a referral to social workers for, which you should be able to find online by searching the name of your country and 'social work assessment for new baby'.

In each country there will be a list of things that midwives **have** to tell social workers about, like if they think you are at risk of domestic abuse.

Your midwife or health professional will tell you if they want to make a social work referral, and will ask for your permission. This is unless they are very worried about your child's safety, and then they can make a referral without you agreeing.

In the UK, social work tends to be divided into two teams: children and adults. If support is being offered for you because you are Autistic, you should have an adult social work assessment. This doesn't always happen, and it can be that a children's social worker does the assessment. You might also have a children's and adult's assessment with two separate social workers and two separate reports.

What happens in a social work assessment?

What is covered in these appointments can vary depending on the country you are in.

These assessments can happen **before you give birth** or may happen after you've given birth.

A social worker will ask you questions about:

- your child's needs
- how you are able to meet their needs
- any needs you can't meet, and who helps you with them.

After the assessment:

- They will then write a report.
- Social workers can't take your baby away from you.
- If a social worker thinks there is a risk of future **significant harm** to your baby, they may ask the court to decide if it would be best for somebody else to be the primary carer for your baby.
- If a social worker thinks there's a risk of **immediate significant harm** to your baby, they would have to contact

the police, and the court process would be done more quickly.

You can watch an Autistic social worker talk about social work assessments and your rights here:

An Autistic midwife's top tips... on looking after baby
By Rebecca Warboys, RM, IBCLC

- Using a sling can help you keep a baby close, but do not fall asleep with your baby in the sling.
- When changing your baby's nappy on a changing station, always keep yourself between them and the floor, even if you haven't seen them roll over yet.
- When changing baby's nappy, don't use cotton wool balls to clean them. The small surface area makes it very hard to use and you need lots. Get cotton wool pads with a bigger surface area if you can.
- When changing a nappy there are differences in how you clean boys and girls. For girls, gently part the outer labia and gently wipe down the vulva front to back. For boys, do not try and clean behind the foreskin – it does not move until boys are around five years old.
- The first time you use a new nappy cream, test it on a small area on baby's bottom in case their skin is sensitive to it.
- Only use a thin layer of nappy cream if you decide to use it, otherwise it will make the inside of the nappy waterproof, and stop it from absorbing pee, which will make nappy rash worse.
- When giving baby a bath, get everything ready before bath time, including two baby bath towels, two nappies (always good to have one ready to mop up any accidents) and their clothes for after the bath.

Conclusion

You've made it to the end of another chapter! We've covered a lot of different things you might experience when caring for a new baby – including safely holding your baby, and managing their toileting, clothes and bathing. We then thought about differences in how some Autistic people parent their child, and that these aren't anything wrong. Finally, I talked about social work assessments. As always, if you're worried about anything, please speak to your GP or health professional. Next, we'll talk about your emotions and mental health with a new baby, although it's OK for you to go to whatever section you like.

CHAPTER 13

Being a New Parent, Emotions and Mental Health

CONTENTS

Introduction

It's completely normal to feel a whole range of negative things, alongside the good things, when you become a new parent. People often don't show this side of parenting, so many parents then feel isolated. In this chapter we'll talk about some common issues.

First, we'll think about your mental health, including 'baby blues', depression, anxiety, Autistic burnout and psychosis. We'll also think about traumatic births and PTSD.

Looking after a new baby almost always means a big change to your situation, with sensory issues and exhaustion as well as not being able to keep to your normal routines.

This change can lead to Autistic burnout. It can be hard to tell if you have depression or burnout. This chapter talks about the differences between these, and when to seek help from a health professional.

Last, we talk about postnatal psychosis (also known as postpartum psychosis or puerperal psychosis), which is less common, but can be very scary when it happens.

There is a lot of difficult content in this chapter, so please do feel free to skip anything, or to come back to this at a later time.

Hormonal shifts after birth, the 'baby blues', depression and anxiety

It's common for most people (Autistic or not) to feel some mixed emotions after they've given birth. Your body has gone through an extremely big change, but that's not the only thing that's going on.

The first week: the 'baby blues'

When you give birth, your hormones change very quickly. In the first week, most people (8 out of 10) have the 'baby blues'. The baby blues usually starts about three or four days after you give birth and should only last a few days.

? **What are the 'baby blues'?**

The feeling of low mood in the **first week** after birth is sometimes called the 'baby blues'. You might:

- feel emotional and cry without a reason
- feel irritated by things that don't usually bother you
- get hot flushes, which are commonly seen during menopause.

! The baby blues should only last a few days.

Hormones and mental health after the first week

Around three or four weeks after you give birth, your hormones will change again. This can impact mental health. It can take up to six months for your hormones to stabilize after you've given birth, and this is a time when you are more likely than normal to have mental health problems.

Up to one in every five people who have given birth will have mental health problems, like anxiety or depression, during pregnancy or after birth.

If you have had anxiety or depression before or during pregnancy, you are more likely to have it after birth. Because Autistic people are more likely to have anxiety and depression, we may be more likely to have it after birth. This doesn't mean all Autistic people will have difficulties with their mental health, but it's good to know this so you can look out for the signs and get help sooner if you need it.

! If you've had mental health problems before, you're more likely to have them again after birth, but that doesn't mean it will happen to you.

If you are already being seen by a health professional for your mental health, you should let them know you are pregnant as soon as possible. It's also important to keep in contact with them, because the hormone changes and change in routine may impact your mental health. Also, your medication may need to be adjusted.

It can be hard to notice changes in your own mental health. That means it might be helpful to ask someone who you trust and know well if they've noticed any changes.

Also, it can be really hard to tell if what you are going through is the usual ups and downs of new parenthood or if you have depression or anxiety. If you have any worries, contact a health professional.

! If you are feeling down or depressed for longer than a week after birth, speak to a health professional like your usual doctor or midwife and ask for help.

? **What is postnatal depression (depression after birth)?**

Postnatal depression can:

- start after birth, but it might also start later in the first year after birth
- come on gradually, or (sometimes very) suddenly
- stop you being able to do the usual activities.

Postnatal depression can include:

- not being interested in or enjoying things you used to
- feeling hopeless, or like you can't cope
- not being able to stop crying
- feeling anxious, very tired or unwell
- not being able to sleep
- not being hungry
- scary thoughts ('intrusive thoughts')
- suicidal thoughts, like 'I want to make this stop'
- suicidal ideation, like 'I'm planning to make this stop by...'

Postnatal depression is usually tested by asking you some questions about your mood. Often the questions are from a tool called the Edinburgh Postnatal Depression Scale.

Suicidal thoughts are when you think things like 'I want to make all of this stop' or 'I wish I could go to bed and just not wake up again.'

Suicidal ideation is different to this. It is thinking about **how** you could kill yourself. This can be having a very clear plan of what you would do. If you find yourself having these thoughts, this is a mental health emergency, and it is **urgent** that you talk to somebody you trust about this. This could be a partner, friend or family member. If you find yourself continuing to think of suicide plans, you should contact your doctor or another health professional for help.

If you find yourself thinking about **how** you could kill yourself ('suicidal ideation'), it is very important to talk to somebody about this **as soon as possible.**

What is postnatal anxiety (anxiety after birth)?

Most new parents will feel worried about looking after their baby.

These thoughts usually get less over time, and are usually gone after a few months.

Postnatal anxiety (anxiety after birth) can include:

- feeling uneasy, worried or scared
- feeling unable to relax and always being on the lookout for bad things
- panic attacks
- avoiding things that remind you of the trauma
- frequent or unstoppable thoughts that stop you being able to live a normal life:
  - The thoughts can get more frequent over time.
  - They can be about things like your baby being sick, something bad happening to your baby, or you not wanting to, but doing something bad to your baby.

Being this anxious can:

- make you feel depressed (see 'What is postnatal depression?', page 318)
- lead to you developing rituals that make you feel less anxious, which can become obsessive compulsive disorder (OCD).

If your health professional thinks you may have postnatal depression or anxiety, they might suggest these treatment options:

- Checking that there isn't a physical cause, like a problem with your thyroid or being anaemic after giving birth. These problems can be easily treated with breastfeeding-safe medication if they are found.

- Getting help from friends and family, so you can spend more time doing things you enjoy and get more sleep, or talking to them about how you are feeling.
- Therapy – like seeing a counsellor or cognitive behavioural therapy.
- Medication – many anti-depressant medications are safe to use when you're breastfeeding, but ask your doctor to check for you.

There may also be peer support for Autistic parents available – in the UK, Autistic Parents UK provides peer support. Social media can also be a way to find groups of Autistic parents.

If these options aren't enough to make you feel better, your doctor can refer you to the perinatal mental health team.

? What is the perinatal mental health team?

There are special teams in each area that focus only on mental health during pregnancy and in the first year after birth. They include mental health nurses, midwives, therapists and doctors (psychiatrists).

They are **experts** in this time and may be able to offer you extra treatment that your usual doctor can't.

Unless your mental health is very severe, you will usually have appointments and go home between these.

If you are extremely unwell, they might have you stay in hospital or a mental health unit until you are a bit better.

If you stay in hospital, this will sometimes be in a special 'mother and baby' mental health unit, where your baby can stay with you. If there isn't space in one of these units, you may be admitted to a regular mental health ward or unit.

It can be hard to know if you are experiencing the usual 'baby blues', postnatal depression, anxiety or Autistic burnout. If you have any worries, seek help from your maternity health professionals or your doctor.

You can watch an Autistic antenatal educator talk about the differences between postnatal depression and Autistic burnout here:

If you are feeling low in mood or very worried about things, speak to a health professional like your usual doctor or midwife and ask for help.

What Autistic people said... about their mental health after birth

- Before giving birth, some people set up appointments with their therapist for after birth to get support in place.
- Being extremely tired was common.
- Some parents didn't always know if they were 'just' exhausted, or if it was depression or burnout.
- Some parents really strongly felt the shift in their mood due to hormones, known as the 'baby blues', but it didn't go away (meaning it became postnatal depression).
- Those who had suicidal ideation (thoughts of how to kill themselves) found it very frightening.
- Those who already had mental health challenges before pregnancy found that pregnancy hormones could make them feel less good than they had before, even if they were still taking medication.
- After birth, some people needed treatment in hospital to stabilize their mental health with medication.
- Postnatal depression could be difficult to treat, with some people needing to try several different medications, and feeling really unwell for a while.
- Those with birth trauma could feel the effects for a very long time afterwards (including future pregnancies).

I don't know what I feel

In Chapter 2 (page 26), we talked about alexithymia. This means not knowing what emotion you are feeling, and it is more common in Autistic people than non-Autistic people.

After birth, you may know that you don't feel right, but might find it hard to know **why** or what emotion you are feeling.

Sometimes giving yourself some time to think can be what you need to work out what is wrong. If you are already overwhelmed or can't get that thinking time this can make it really difficult.

You might want to look at the questions below to help you think about your feelings. I've also included signs of pain and infection, because Autistic people aren't always good at knowing when something is physically wrong with ourselves.

Tool: Checklist for when you don't feel right after birth

Are you in pain or might you have an infection?

Think specifically, do you have:

- pain low down in your tummy (lower abdomen)?
- any pain, redness or heat in either breast?
- redness, discharge or swelling around your C-section incision or stitches?
- blood loss from your vagina?
- a really bad-smelling discharge from your vagina?
- a high or low temperature?
- a headache?

Are your basic needs met?

When did you last:

- have a drink?
- eat?
- sleep?
- go to the toilet to pee or poo?
- do something you find calming, even if only for a few minutes?

Is something else bothering you?

Do you feel:

- dysregulated? – you could try some of the things that help you self-regulate: see the tools in Chapter 2, pages 32 and 34
- overwhelmed – is there anyone you trust who you could ask to help with your baby, to give you some rest?
- irritated by something somebody has done – you could try getting it out, say by talking to someone, talking to yourself, or writing down your thoughts.

Birth trauma

Even a straightforward birth can leave people with birth trauma. It is more likely if you needed emergency treatment, like an unplanned C-section or other interventions from doctors, or a long or painful birth.

Having a difficult birth is known to make it more likely that you will have mental health problems. This can include developing post-traumatic stress disorder (PTSD) and finding it difficult to bond with your baby.

Autistic people are more likely to have PTSD than non-Autistic people.

What is post-traumatic stress disorder (PTSD)?

PTSD, or post-traumatic stress disorder, is a type of anxiety disorder that can happen when you go through a very difficult event.

These events can include a difficult birth, being violently or sexually assaulted or being involved in a war or natural disaster.

PTSD can include:

- reliving the trauma, including 'flashbacks' or nightmares
- avoiding things that you think may trigger you
- finding it difficult to sleep
- these things having a big impact on your day-to-day activities.

If you have experienced a lot of traumatic situations, especially in childhood, you can get **complex PTSD** (or C-PTSD).

C-PTSD can include:

- feeling shame or guilt about what happened
- feeling worthless
- finding it hard to control your emotions.

If you are still having problems because of birth trauma a month after you give birth, seek advice from your doctor or health professional.

Treatments for birth trauma, including if it leads to PTSD or C-PTSD, are:

- an appointment with a midwife to discuss what happened – some people say this makes them feel better
- taking medication (anti-depressants) – many are safe when breastfeeding
- therapy, particularly trauma-based approaches and eye movement desensitization and reprocessing (EMDR).

Small or unwell babies

If your baby is small, also called 'low birthweight', they may need to stay in hospital for extra monitoring and treatment. This isn't optional; if the doctors think baby is too poorly to go home, they can insist that baby stays.

Having a baby that needs to stay in hospital for longer than usual can be hard for any parent. It may be even harder for Autistic parents to cope with the uncertainty, and the sensory environment when they are in hospital with baby. This can include having to sit (and sleep sometimes) in uncomfortable chairs, bright lights and lots of noise, including frequent alarms going off.

You can watch an Autistic parent talk about:

- their experience of giving birth to a small baby and them needing to stay in hospital here:
- having a baby on the special care baby unit here:

Sensory changes, exhaustion, changes to your routine and lack of control

New parenthood is a lot for anybody. Many Autistic people will have carefully controlled their life to keep them feeling well. A new baby can mean big changes to those routines **and** new sensory experiences, which can be really difficult.

What Autistic people said... about challenges of being a new parent

- Baby's crying could be really painful, which made some parents feel like bad parents.
- One way of coping with the pain of baby crying was to put them somewhere safe and either take a few minutes to re-regulate or ask for help from other adults in the home.
- Having disrupted sleep and not enough sleep was one of the hardest thing for many.
- In the early weeks, constantly needing to feed baby (whether by breast or bottle) was a lot; knowing it got easier after around six weeks really helped.
- In the early weeks, it's hard to know what baby needs and there isn't really any kind of routine.

- It's hard to know if you're 'just' exhausted or if it's postnatal depression.
- It can be hard to co-parent: partners might not do the things they said they would.
- Bringing a second (or third or fourth) baby into a home could be much more difficult than the first, as older children could be dysregulated and demanding.

You can watch an Autistic antenatal educator talk about some of the sensory challenges in early parenthood here:

Some Autistic parents found the intensity of touch when caring for a new baby hard. This is sometimes called being 'touched out'. Some parents found wearing extra layers of clothes could reduce the impact of this. If they were breastfeeding wearing two tops and pulling one up and the other down reduced how much bare skin was exposed.

It's always OK to put your baby down somewhere safe and have a break if you need to.

Some Autistic parents can find it hard to recognize their baby. This can be not being able to recognize your baby's face, which is sometimes called 'face blindness' (or prosopagnosia), or their smell. Try not to worry if this happens to you – over time you will come to recognize your baby in some other way.

You can watch an Autistic parent talk about their experience of 'face blindness' (prosopagnosia) here:

You may find yourself feeling a lot of pressure to be the perfect parent. This could be always doing something, like keeping your home clean and tidy to your usual standard. Most parents would struggle to do this, so it might be best to let your standards slip for a while.

One way of relaxing your standards is to have a postnatal 'babymoon'. Babymoons aren't a new thing and lots of cultures support new birthing parents to relax and recover after birth.

What is a postnatal babymoon?

A babymoon has two meanings: a holiday before you give birth **and** relaxed time alone with your baby after you give birth.

We're thinking about the second meaning here.

A postnatal babymoon is time when you, your baby and your partner/chosen supporters spend relaxed, uninterrupted time together. This means the normal rules don't apply.

People who have a babymoon:

- meet their baby's needs, including cuddling, feeding, changing their nappies and sleeping...and repeat
- bond with their baby by spending lots of relaxed time being together – if you enjoy skin-to-skin with your baby, you can do plenty of this
- keep themself fed and drinking enough (especially if breastfeeding)
- sleep and rest as much as possible
- put off all but essential tasks – not worrying about housework beyond the essentials, like sterilizing bottles if they're using them, having a clean space in your kitchen if they're formula feeding, and doing baby's washing
- only allow people to visit if they really want them to
- ask trusted people to help, such as by bringing meals, doing shopping for them and helping out in their home, like doing laundry or dishes.

Script: Telling people you're having a babymoon (after baby is born)

- 'We're having a babymoon; it's like a honeymoon so only me, (partner) and baby for the first few weeks. It's got lots of benefits for the baby.'
- 'I'm hoping to breastfeed, and one thing that helps is having a "babymoon". It means you have relaxed time alone as a family and no visitors.'
- 'Thanks for offering to help. We're having a babymoon, which means we aren't having people see me or meet the baby yet. If you'd still like to help, we'd appreciate it if you could cook a dinner for us or come around and clean the kitchen, but it's completely OK if you don't want to do that.'
- 'Sorry, we're not having visitors for the first month, we're having a babymoon.'

Autistic burnout

As well as mental health conditions, another thing that can impact Autistic parents is Autistic burnout.

Autistic burnout happens when our needs are not met consistently over a period of time.

Needing to look after a new baby is a time when all parents have to put their needs aside to an extent.

You can watch an Autistic NICU (neonatal intensive care unit) nurse talk about spotting the signs of depression and/or Autistic burnout in maternity here:

What Autistic people said... about Autistic burnout when parenting

- They often knew the things that were taking too much energy, but tried to push through.
- Things that could take too much energy included:
  - too many visitors (especially the unhelpful ones)
  - going out (especially to doctors appointments or shopping) when already feel overwhelmed
  - not going outside when they found being outside energizing
  - doing more than essential housework.
- Burnout could be like:
  - feeling 'drained' or 'exhausted' even when they got a lot of sleep
  - everything feeling like a 'blur' or like you weren't really there.
- Things that helped included:
  - knowing it's normal for babies not to sleep through the night
  - getting help and learning not to feel bad about this; those with a partner sometimes took 'shifts' to get more sleep
  - safely co-sleeping (see Chapter 11, page 266 for more information)
  - wearing their baby in a sling or carrier.

You can watch an Autistic parent talk about their experiences of overwhelm after birth, including becoming non-speaking, here:

These massive changes can also impact partners who are co-parenting with you. They would need to seek help from their own doctor.

You can watch an Autistic dad talk about his experiences of postnatal depression, burnout and returning to work here:

Postnatal psychosis

Psychosis after you've given birth is rarer than depression and anxiety, impacting around 1 in 1000 people who give birth.

If you have bipolar type 1 or schizoaffective disorder, or previously had postnatal psychosis, you have at least a 1 in 10 (10%) chance of getting postnatal psychosis.

If you have a blood-relative who had postnatal psychosis, you are also more likely to get it. But it can happen to anyone, even if you have never had a mental health issue before.

Postnatal psychosis usually starts in the first two weeks after birth, but can happen later. It is very serious, as it makes it difficult for you to look after yourself and your baby.

If you have postnatal psychosis, you would **suddenly** get some or all of these things (or 'symptoms'):

- Mania – this means feeling 'high' or 'manic', like you're 'on top of the world'.
- Depression – this means being low in mood, tearful or anxious.
- Very quick changes in your mood from being 'high' to 'low'.
- Feeling very confused.
- Hallucinations – this means seeing, hearing, smelling, touching or tasting things that aren't there, or thinking something happened that didn't.
- Having odd thoughts or delusions – this means strongly believing something that isn't true. Sometimes this could be that your baby is possessed by the devil.
- Paranoia – this is when you continuously think people are 'out to get you' even though nothing has happened to make you think this. It can make you feel very scared, including of other people.

- Racing thoughts.
- Behaving in a way you wouldn't usually, including being more 'free' (or disinhibited) than usual.

The symptoms can change very quickly – even within an hour or two.

It is common for people with postnatal psychosis to not know or believe they are ill. This means that the people around them usually spot the changes and have to help them get help.

! Postnatal psychosis is rare, but it is a mental health emergency than needs urgent treatment.

Talking to health professionals

Throughout this chapter I've said lots of times to talk to your health professional if you have any worries.

Many Autistic people find it difficult to set up appointments or to raise difficult topics.

In the UK, there is usually a check-up for all new parents and babies on day 5. The programme of check-ups may be different in other countries, so ask your midwife or health professional if you don't know what will be offered. If you are having any worries at all about your mental health – even if they are small – please tell them during the check. If you forget or aren't able to tell them then, it's OK to tell your midwife or doctor at any other time.

? What happens at the day 5 postnatal (after birth) check?

- Baby can have a blood test for serious health conditions, like cystic fibrosis. They do this by pricking baby's heel and collecting a few drops of blood on a special card. You can feed or cuddle baby when they do this to reduce the pain they feel.
- Baby will usually be weighed naked (without a nappy). It's usually considered normal for them to lose up to 10 per cent of their weight from when they were born.

- If baby has lost more than about 8 per cent of their birthweight, they will make a plan to make sure feeding is going well and to make sure baby gains weight.
- They will look at the baby's head and body to check everything looks OK, including their cord stump (belly button).
- They will ask you about feeding, and the number of wet and dirty nappies baby has. This is the time to tell them if you have any worries about breast or formula feeding, including if you have any breast pain, redness or hot skin.
- They will ask you about any incisions or stitches and how they are feeling. This is the time to tell them if you're having any pain, discharge or bleeding.
- They may ask you about your mental health. If they don't ask the question, it's still important to tell them if you're not feeling well with your mental health.
- If you have any other worries about yourself or baby, this is a good time to ask the midwife or health professional about them.

Script: Some things it might be helpful to say to a health professional if you're worried about you or baby

Tell them about the problem, for example:

- 'I don't think baby is feeding enough.'
- 'Baby isn't having any dirty (poo) nappies.'
- 'Baby seems very tired and isn't alert when awake.'
- 'My breasts/nipples hurt.'
- 'I feel unwell and think I might have an infection.'
- 'My mood is very low and I'm worried about it.'

Tell them how long it's been going on:

- 'I've been like this for (say a number) of days.'
- 'It started on (say the first day, e.g. Tuesday).'

You might want to tell them you're Autistic and if you think that could be impacting things or making them more serious:

- 'Because I'm Autistic, I can't tell if there's a problem with how I'm breastfeeding.'
- 'Because I'm Autistic, I'm at greater risk for postnatal depression.'

You can watch an Autistic maternity support worker talk about the day 5 check-up here:

An Autistic midwife's top tips... on emotions and mental health after birth
By Rebecca Warboys, RM, IBCLC

- If you are experiencing the baby blues I find it is helpful to consider it like a wave that will come and go; when you feel low, knowing you will feel better again really helps. Rest and do what you need to do to help yourself feel a little better again.
- If you struggle to recognize your baby, you can use baby's clothing, sounds or smell to help you start to build recognition.
- If you experience psychosis after the birth of your baby, this is nothing you have done wrong and you do not need to be ashamed. You can get help. It does not mean your baby will be taken away if you admit these feelings, but just that you will get help to feel better and keep your baby safe.
- There is some evidence that if you have experienced a traumatic event (like a birth you found traumatic), playing a game like Tetris on your phone within six hours after the event can help reduce the trauma later on.

- Make some meal batches and freeze them when still pregnant. You can use these for familiar meals after baby is born and reduce the pressure to cook.

Conclusion

You've made it to the end of another chapter! We've covered a lot of different things you might experience in new parenting – including a lot of increased sensory input like crying and the baby touching you a lot, as well as the reduced ability to sleep and rest. We've also talked about the emotions, mental health and Autistic burnout that can go alongside these big changes. I've also talked about some of the ways that you might be able to tell if you need to ask for help with your mental health. I hope this gives you some reassurance, but if you're worried about anything, please speak to your GP or health professional. Next, we'll go to the conclusion of the book, although it's OK for you to go to whatever section you like and to skip the conclusion (there isn't any new information).

CHAPTER 14

Conclusion

There are so many different options and things that can happen by chance when it comes to maternity. When you are Autistic and pregnant (or a new parent) there may be even more different and unexpected things.

I hope this book has been – or will be – useful for you in knowing about some of these.

We've heard lots of different experiences from Autistic parents in the book, which I hope are helpful or reassuring. At the moment, we don't know very much about Autistic people's pregnancy experiences, so if something different happens to you or you feel something different, that doesn't mean you're wrong.

The key point is:

! If you're not sure about something, ask for help. Health professionals and breastfeeding supporters are there to help you.

Some other important points from the book are:

Chapter 2: sensory

- Autistic people can feel some senses too much, which can cause pain, and some things not enough. This can get bigger in pregnancy. It is helpful to know what things are difficult for you, so you can try to change the environment.
- Many Autistic people experience pain differently to non-Autistic people. It might be helpful to think about how you feel pain

so you can tell your birthing partner and health professionals before birth.

Chapter 3: staying healthy

- There are medicines that can be taken to reduce nausea in pregnancy, so if you're struggling to eat or drink, contact your midwife or GP.
- Any bleeding in pregnancy is cause for concern, and you should get checked by your midwife, doctor or local maternity unit. Don't wait for your next appointment; phone them straight away.

Chapter 4: maternity appointments

- You have the right to say no to any treatment or tests at any time.
- Being Autistic means that you have the right in many countries to ask for changes to make healthcare easier for you to access ('disability accommodations').

Chapter 5: finding information and supportive people

- You don't have to listen to people around you when they are giving their views on your pregnancy.
- News sites and social media often aren't good sources of information about pregnancy – look at the health agency for your country instead.

Chapter 6: pregnancy complications and loss

- If you are worried about your pregnancy, don't wait until the next appointment; phone your midwife or local maternity unit. They are open day and night.
- It's important to know your baby's pattern of movements. If your baby's movements slow down, stop or change, phone your

local maternity unit as soon as possible, as your baby could be unwell – it can be life threatening.

- If you have a pregnancy loss be very kind to yourself; most pregnancy losses cannot be prevented.

Chapter 7: changes shortly before birth

- When your waters break, it can be a trickle, rather than the dramatic gushing you see on TV shows. If you think your waters have broken, phone your maternity unit, as baby has more risk of getting an infection after your waters break.

Chapter 8: where to give birth

- You get to decide where you want to give birth. The health professionals can only make suggestions. The pain relief options vary depending on where you give birth. For example, doctors are needed to give an epidural, but there may not be birthing pools on doctor-led birthing wards.
- You get to decide who is with you when you give birth, including a birthing partner, and if you'd be happy to have student midwives and doctors in the room.

Chapter 9: stages of birth and pain relief

- If baby's heart rate slows down (they 'become distressed') it is an emergency and they need to be born quickly by having a C-section or forceps birth.
- During labour, it's OK to use a range of ways to reduce pain. You might want to use your breathing, have your birthing partner massage you, move your body or make noises, as well as trying hypnobirthing, a TENS machine or using medication.
- If you want an epidural, you should ask for this early in labour, as it might take a while for the doctor to be free to see you, and it takes up to 40 minutes to work.

Chapter 10: immediately after birth

- It's helpful for you to decide before you give birth if you want baby to have delayed cord clamping or a vitamin K injection, if you want an injection to help deliver the placenta, and if you want to do 'skin-to-skin' with baby. Tell your birthing partner or midwife your decisions ahead of time so they can help you get the care you want.
- After birth you will be asked to have an examination of your genitals to see if you have any injuries from birth ('tears'). You may be offered stitches if the tear is bleeding or includes your anus.

Chapter 11: sleep, crying and feeding

- It's really important to follow safer sleeping advice, including not sleeping with baby on a sofa or armchair. This is because babies are at risk of suddenly dying without a clear reason (known as sudden infant death syndrome or SIDS).
- Babies can cry a lot. You might want to create a 'checklist' of things you run through to try to soothe them.
- Newborn babies have very small tummies, so it's normal for them to need to feed about 12 times a day.

Chapter 12: caring for baby

- If you aren't sure how to do any part of looking after your baby, the UK NHS website has detailed information and videos. You can also ask your health professional.
- There is no single right way to look after and connect with your baby, and no evidence that Autistic parents are worse than non-Autistic parents.

Chapter 13: emotions and mental health

- Most parents (4 in 5) get the 'baby blues' after giving birth. This is when you have a low mood. It should only last a few days; speak to your midwife or doctor if it lasts longer.

- If you find yourself thinking about how you could kill yourself ('suicidal ideation') this is a mental health emergency, and you should tell someone you trust as soon as possible, and speak to your midwife or doctor urgently.

Thank you for reading this book.

If you have any feedback, you can contact me on Blue Sky: @DrAimeeGrant, or via Jessica Kingsley Publishers.

Useful Resources

Autistic maternity

Autistic and Expecting: Practical Support for Parents-to-Be and Health and Social Care Practitioners by Alexis Quinn: This is a more in-depth guide to pregnancy for Autistic people. Chapter 1 has good information on your rights in pregnancy and getting reasonable adjustments during maternity care.

Supporting Autistic People Through Pregnancy and Childbirth by Hayley Morgan and colleagues: This book is an advanced read that explores lots of research on pregnancy for Autistic people.

From Here to Maternity: Pregnancy and Motherhood on the Autism by Lana Grant: One Autistic person's detailed description of their different maternity journeys when having their children.

The Autistic Pregnancy Birth and Beyond: Your Questions Answered: A collection of 114 short videos by Autistic parents and Autistic maternity professionals (UK context). www.swansea.ac.uk/research/research-highlights/health-innovation/Autistic-pregnancy-birth-and-beyond

Also available via:
www.youtube.com/@AutismMenstruationToMenopause

Staying well when you're Autistic (not pregnancy specific) - Chapter 2

Looking After Your Autistic Self: A Personalised Self-Care Approach to Managing Your Sensory and Emotional Well-Being by Niamh Garvey

Taking Off the Mask: Practical Exercises to Help Understand and Minimise the Effects of Autistic Camouflaging by Hannah Belcher (especially Chapter 5)

Finding good quality information about maternity – Chapter 5

Informed Is Best: How to Spot Fake News About Your Pregnancy, Birth and Baby by Amy Brown

Pregnancy loss – Chapter 6

Coping With Pregnancy Loss by Petra Boynton

Tommy's: Pregnancy loss charity
www.tommys.org

Planning your birth – Chapters 8, 9 and 10

BRAIN: A tool to help make decisions about treatment for you and your baby (can be used as a template to ask for more information)
www.liverpoolwomens.nhs.uk/our-services/maternity/your-antenatal-care/brain

Birthrights: A charity focused on rights during pregnancy and birth
https://birthrights.org.uk

Feeding baby – Chapter 11

The Positive Breastfeeding Book: Everything You Need to Feed Your Baby with Confidence by Amy Brown

Guest Blog: 'Is This Normal?': Blog by Emma Pickett for UNICEF's Baby Friendly Initiative
www.unicef.org.uk/babyfriendly/is-this-normal

KellyMom: A website developed by a mother of three who is also an International Board Certified Lactation Consultant (IBCLC) to provide information on breastfeeding and parenting.
www.Kellymom.com

Index